To: James Buchanan
with warm
regards

John C Goodman

NATIONAL HEALTH CARE IN GREAT BRITAIN: LESSONS FOR THE U.S.A.

John C. Goodman, Ph.D
University of Dallas

A FISHER INSTITUTE PUBLICATION

ISBN: 0-933028-04-0 (paperback)
ISBN: 0-933028-05-9 (hardcover)

Library of Congress Catalogue Number 79-55246

Printed in the United States of America

ABOUT THE AUTHOR

Dr. John Goodman is currently an assistant professor in the Department of Economics at the University of Dallas. However, his teaching and publishing career has taken him to teaching assignments at the University of Texas at Austin, Sarah Lawrence College, Columbia University, Dartmouth College and Southern Methodist University.

After receiving his Ph.D. from Columbia, Dr. Goodman published several articles in the areas of his special interest: public choice, industrial organization and the economics of regulation.

This will mark his third book publishing effort. His previous books have included *Economics of Public Policy: the Micro View* (with Ed Dolan) and *Opting Out of Social Security in Great Britain* (for the American Enterprise Institute). Dr. Goodman has been awarded fellowships by the National Endowment for the Humanities and the Hoover Institution at Stanford University.

ACKNOWLEDGMENTS

For their assistance in gathering the most up-to-date information available about the National Health Service and other health care statistics in Great Britain, the author is indebted to Arthur Seldon and John Wood of the Institute of Economic Affairs, John Ford of the British Medical Association, Dianna Scarrott of the British Dental Association, Brian Bricknell of the British United Provident Association, Jeremy Hurst of the Department of Health and Social Security, and David Taylor of the Office of Health Economics.

The author also acknowledges the valuable assistance provided by the following U.S. individuals and organizations: Stuart Butler of The Heritage Foundation (Washington, DC), Laura Reesby of the Harris County Medical Society (Houston, TX), Dr. Joseph M. Merrill of the Baylor College of Medicine (Houston, TX), and Max Horlick and other members of the staff of the International Division of the Office of Research and Statistics, Social Security Administration. The views expressed in this publication are those of the author, and do not necessarily reflect the views of those individuals listed above.

The author would also like to express special appreciation to Susan M. Tully, without whose help this book would not have been published, and to Bridgett Gaines, who also assisted in the preparation of the manuscript. Appreciation is also extended to The Fisher Institute (Dallas, TX) for financial assistance and the editing of the original manuscript.

TABLE OF CONTENTS

1. **Introduction**   1

2. **Historical Background**   5
   The Poor Law
   Private Charity and Mutual Aid
   The National Health Insurance Act of 1911
   Prelude to the National Health Service
   The National Health Service White Paper, 1944
   The National Health Service Act, 1946

3. **The Organization of British Health Care Today**   19
   Administrative Structure
   The Budgetary Costs of the N.H.S.

4. **The National Health Service and Some General**   29
   Principles of Health Economics
   Is Health Care Different?
   Medical "Need" Versus Medical "Demand"
   Health Care and Life Expectancy
   Health Care and Economic Efficiency

5. **Rationing: The General Practitioner**   55
   The Role of the Family Doctor
   Who Demands Care?
   The Supply of General Practitioner Services
   The Financial Incentives of General Practitioners
   Financial Incentives and Other Aspects of
    General Practice
   The Alternatives Open to Patients
   Who Receives Care?
   Economic Efficiency in General Practice

6. **Rationing: The Hospital Sector**   89
   The Waiting Lists
   The Demand for Hospital Services
   The Supply of Hospital Care
   The Quality of Care: Hospital Incentives
   The Quality of Care: Doctor Incentives
   The Quality of Care: Incentives of Hospital
    Workers

What Can Patients Do?
Who Receives Care?
Economic Efficiency in the Hospital Sector

7. **Rationing: Other N.H.S. Sectors**   **143**
   Community Health and "Other" Services
   General Dental Services
   Ophthalmic Services
   Pharmaceutical Services

8. **The Trend Toward Private Care**   **161**
   General Practitioners
   N.H.S. Hospitals
   Private Hospitals and Nursing Homes
   Private Health Insurance

9. **Inequalities in the National Health Service**   **175**
   Inequality: Geography and Medical Need
   Inequality: The Role of Social Class

10. **The Politics of Medicine**   **185**
    Public Choice Theory
    The Total Amount of Spending on Health
      Services
    Inequalities in the National Health Service
    Spending Priorities: "Caring" Versus "Curing"
    Spending Priorities: Current Expenditure Versus
      Capital Expenditure
    Administrative Controls
    Why the N.H.S. Continues to Exist

11. **Lessons for the U.S.A.**   **207**

Chapter 1
Introduction

By most accounts, Britain is the most socialistic of all the western industrial democracies. It is *not* particularly socialistic in terms of having achieved a more equal distribution of income and wealth. The true distribution of income in Great Britain is probably not much different from that exhibited in the United States. The distribution of wealth in Britain is probably *more* unequal than its distribution in the United States. But Britain *is* socialistic in terms of having transferred to the state more and more power over economic resources.

In recent years, over 60 percent of Britain's national income has been spent through the government. Its tax rates on income and wealth are among the highest in the world. One-third of the British labor force works for the government. One-third of British families live in houses owned and operated by the state.

The British are also socialistic in terms of attitude. There is a widespread antipathy toward competition in the marketplace. Government subsidies and loans to business are now so large and diverse that no one has the foggiest idea which enterprises would succeed or which would fail if gains and losses were determined by the free market. No firm or industry falters, far less fails, without immediate application for succor from the state. While the British are quick to reward failure, success is almost universally despised. Enoch Powell, former Minister of Health, has described Britain as "a country where making a profit is treated as prima facia calling for apology."

Many of the failures of British socialism are well known. Since 1970, Britain has recorded the highest inflation rate, the lowest rate of economic growth, and smallest increase in worker productivity among major industrialized countries. Less than 20 years ago, the British standard of living was superior to that in most European countries, including West Germany. Today, private consumption expenditure per person (a handy measure of well-being) in Britain is about half that in Switzerland, West Germany and France, and not much more than that of Italy and Spain. By some measurements, Britain is now a poorer country than East Germany.

It should come as no surprise to learn that in a country where making a profit calls for an apology, "profiting on sickness" is regarded as the worst of entrepreneurial sins. The British have gone a long way toward removing the temptation to commit such sins with a comprehensive system of socialized medicine. Yet, while most of Britain's failures are widely recognized, the failures of socialized medicine, British style, are not generally known.

In fact, it was not so long ago that the British system of socialized medicine was hailed as a system that America should emulate. The British, it was said, had proved that socialized medicine works — and works well. In 1978, Joseph Califano, then Secretary of Health, Education and Welfare, bestowed lavish praise on the British National Health Service during a visit to England.

Yet the image of the British National Health Service is becoming increasingly tarnished by newspaper headlines ("BRITAIN'S HEALTH SERVICE TO UNDERGO INVESTIGATION"; "BRITISH HOSPITALS HIT BY SLOWDOWN OF YOUNG DOCTORS"), and by the investigative research of Britain's own health economists. British economist Dennis Lees recently summarized the judgment of many when he wrote that "the substitution of socialized medicine for private medicine has not led to *more* medical care; to *better* medical care; or to a more *equal distribution* of medical care. There is in Britain today grave uncertainty about both the availability and quality of medical care." In fact, among the most knowledgeable advocates of socialized medicine, the British system is no longer regarded as the ideal. As often as not these days, advocates of socialized medicine in the United States refer to Britain as the "worst case," and reserve their praise for the systems of other countries.

The British experience with socialized medicine is important, however. It is an experience ripe with lessons for the U.S. In fact, we are likely to learn more about the pitfalls of state-provided medical care from the British case than by studying the health system of just about any other country. This is true for two reasons: First, the British have a more comprehensive system of state-provided medical care than any other western industrial country. Over 95 percent of medical expenditures in Britain flow through the state. Sweden and New Zealand tie for second place with about 80 percent. By studying the British health care system, then, we can be far more confident that we are studying the genuine results of socialized medical care and not the potentially misleading case of a mixed system of public and private medicine.

Second, the British experience is especially instructive precisely because Britain is less wealthy than other nations. Only in recent years have policy-makers in the United States, Sweden, Canada and West Germany fully come face to face with a modern reality: society cannot possibly provide all of its citizens with all that medical science has to offer. The British, with their more limited health care budget, have dealt with this reality for decades. Moreover, it is becoming increasingly evident that other nations are slowly but surely following in Britain's footsteps.

This study is a comprehensive analysis of the British National Health Service. It differs from all previous studies of this system in one crucial respect — it relies on fundamental economic principles. It incorporates not only the traditional tools of economic science, but also the insights of a relatively new branch of economics — public choice theory. Public choice theory attempts to explain public policies which evolve through the political system in much the same way that economists explain behavior in the economic marketplace.

The British health care system has been studied extensively by the British themselves. In general, there has been no reluctance to identify failure. But British studies almost universally share a common theme: major defects and problems in the N.H.S. are regarded as the result of institutional or historical accident. Inevitably such studies suggest that all that is fundamentally lacking is the will to make the system work better.

By contrast, this study attempts to show that most of the problems and defects of the N.H.S. follow logically from fundamental principles governing human behavior. As Enoch Powell has written, most of these defects "are not the accidental or incidental results of blemishes which can be 'reformed' away while leaving the system as such intact." Instead, they are the natural and inevitable consequences of placing health care in the hands of the state.

Economics is a positive science, not a normative one. It cannot tell us what kind of health care system we *ought* to have. The principal finding of this study as it relates to an American health care system is that *any health care system modeled after the British National Health Service would promise very few benefits and very high costs.*

Chapter 2
Historical Background

The National Health Service, established in 1948, was not a radically new policy of the British welfare state. It was the product of evolution, not revolution. Behind it lay centuries of tradition in the provision of health care and the organization of medical practitioners. It was preceded by the National Health Insurance Act of 1911, which provided a form of health insurance for low- and lower-middle-income workers, and by the infamous Poor Law, which governed public welfare policies for centuries.

It is no accident that public provision of medical care has had a long association with public provisions for the relief of poverty. Prior to the twentieth century, the medical profession had very little of value to offer in the marketplace. The general practitioner could often do little more for his patients than comfort and console them. Similarly, hospitals were not primarily instututions devoted to healing — they were places where people went to die.[1]

For those who came to rely on public welfare, then, there was often little distinction made between "care" and "medical care." Indeed, there was rarely any reason to make such a distinction. It is for this reason that the historical origins of socialized medicine in Britain today are to be found in the British policies toward the relief of poverty — policies that were established centuries ago.

The Poor Law

National concern with the problem of poverty was reflected in the much-maligned *Act for the Reliefe of the Poore,* legislated in 1598 during the reign of Elizabeth I. Enacted in 1601, it remained, with some modifications, the law of England until 1948. The Poor Law provided for relief for the elderly and those unable to work by empowering local parishes to collect taxes and to appoint "overseers of the poor."[2] Several provisions of the Law, as amended by 1834, ensured that only those who had no alternative sources of aid sought public relief. The first of these provisions was the *means test.* The family of an applicant for relief was held to have a legal liability for the care and relief of that person if that family possessed adequate financial resources. Beyond the family, the liability fell to the local community in which the applicant lived.

The second provision was the principle of *less eligibility*. This principle stipulated that the conditions of public relief be such that the position of the relieved be kept below that of the poorest independent worker. To that end, recipients of relief were required to live in "poorhouses" if unable to work, and in "workhouses" if "able-bodied" and unemployed. "Unregenerate idlers" were lodged in "houses of correction." Those living on relief had to submit to rules and regulations which today seem quite harsh. Silence was maintained at all meals, families were separated, and alcohol, tobacco and visitors were forbidden. Conditions of the acceptance of relief were such that all but the most destitute ordinarily refused it.

Overall, the poor-law system was quite successful in providing food and shelter for millions of poverty-stricken individuals. Medical care of some sort existed in the public relief houses, and by the end of the eighteenth century most parishes provided some medical services for the poor in their own homes.[3] But the effectiveness of the poor law system varied greatly from parish to parish, and the burden of local taxation was often resented.[4] Concern over taxes was not greatly lessened when an independent Central Board replaced the local parish administration in 1834.

Spurred by a massive cholera epidemic in 1866, Poor Law authorities were convinced that further steps were needed to prevent the spread of disease. The condition of the workhouse sick was widely denounced, and beginning in 1867 parishes were urged to form "Sick Asylum Districts" to support hospitals in which workhouse residents could be treated. This was particularly successful in London, where isolation hospitals for infectious cases, infirmaries for the non-infectious, asylums for the mentally-ill, and dispensaries for outpatients were established. Although intended for paupers, the poor-law hospitals were soon admitting anyone needing treatment, since in many cases no other facilities were available.[5]

Private Charity and Mutual Aid

In addition to public relief, private charity provided medical services to the poor — usually through voluntary hospitals first established by religious institutions. Although such hospitals had existed in previous centuries, their number expanded greatly in the eighteenth century. Between 1720 and 1745, five hospitals were founded in

London. The first, Guy's Hospital, was endowed entirely by one individual. In time, a tradition developed whereby prominent members of the medical profession provided their services free of charge to the voluntary hospitals.[6]

A third option existed for the working class poor, many of whom feared that illness might force them to accept shelter in the poorhouse. Mutual aid groups called *friendly societies* developed, particularly among workers employed in the same occupation. These organizations, which were the forerunners of modern insurance companies, provided sick pay, medical care, and a death benefit to their members in return for weekly contributions. Provisions for medical care normally worked like this: an agreement between a friendly society and a doctor stipulated that, in return for a fixed salary, the doctor would give medical care to society members.[7]

The friendly societies ensured their members some measure of financial independence, and were immensely popular. An estimated four and a half million people belonged to friendly societies in the late nineteenth century — over half the adult male population in Great Britain.[8] But membership was not open to all; in general, only skilled workers were eligible. Some societies accepted only teetotalers, others only members of a certain religious sect. And none provided medical care for women or children.

As the Victorian Age drew to a close, friendly society enrollment remained high, but the organizations were in trouble. The fraternal spirit which had originally characterized such societies vanished as they grew larger. Their most serious difficulties were financial: contribution and benefit rates were based on rapidly outdated actuarial information. Due largely to better living conditions, people were simply living longer. Many societies, not anticipating the large number of sickness claims among their members, found themselves in desperate straits. Some were near bankruptcy. Nonetheless, the friendly societies wielded a great deal of political power, even in their declining years. Their role in shaping the National Health Insurance Act of 1911 was especially important.[9]

The National Health Insurance Act of 1911

In 1911, national health insurance for low- and lower-middle-income workers came to Britain. The legislation is usually regarded as the brainchild of David Lloyd George, Chancellor of the Exchequer under the Liberal Government. Lloyd George was primarily concerned with sickness as a cause of poverty, not for its own sake. His proposal sought to provide medical care for the breadwinner — but not his family — so that he could return to work.

The plan was financed by a weekly tax of fourpence paid by the insured worker, a tax of threepence on the worker's employer, and an additional twopence contribution from the state. In return, insured workers were entitled to receive medical treatment and cash benefits for sickness and disability. The plan also provided for institutional care in sanitoria for cases of tuberculosis and, in some cases, additional benefits for dental and ophthalmic care.[10]

The Lloyd George scheme was sold to the public on the cry of "ninepence for fourpence." In other words, low-income workers were told that they were being offered benefits whose value was more than twice the value of their weekly fourpenny contribution.[11] The facts were otherwise. Both economic theory and empirical evidence suggest that employment taxes are not actually borne by employers. The threepence employer contribution was simply part of the cost of hiring a worker for one week. Employers had no financial reason to care whether the "contribution" went to an insurance scheme or to workers in the form of wages. So most economists believe that the burden of such taxes ultimately falls on the workers themselves. In the absence of the tax, the worker's weekly wage would have been threepence higher. In addition, part of the burden of general taxes undoubtedly fell on low-income workers. So the twopence contribution from the state partly came out of the pockets of workers as well. The siren song of something for nothing, then, was largely a hoax.

The plan also received support from less gullible quarters. By the turn of the century, an important change was taking place in the thinking of a great many members of the educated elite. Increasingly, they began to approve of the use of coercion to force the lower classes to reorder their lives. Paternalism was coming of age and was forming the intellectual foundations for the development of the British welfare state. British writer Colm Brogan has described this type of thinking in the following way:

> Social reformers, most notably the Fabians and, most notably of all, the Webbs,[12] believed that the working class were not fit to look after their own affairs or to provide for their own needs. They were a drinking, gambling, improvident, and irresponsible lot who threw their money around like confetti when times were good and had to appeal for alms when bad times came for which they had made no provision. They were

also a lawless lot requiring the pressures of exterior disciplines. Beatrice Webb believed that if the police were withdrawn from the London streets for twenty-four hours the city would immediately sink into the condition of the Congo on a particularly bad day. Considering the ignorance and fecklessness of the working class, it was good policy not only to provide what they were unable to pay but also to extract from them what they were unwilling to pay. Beatrice Webb saw herself as a mother who gently but firmly puts away some of her child's pocket money, and there were many of the same mind.[13]

To make the plan workable, Lloyd George needed the political support of the friendly societies and the cooperation of commercial insurance companies and the doctors. He achieved these goals through skillful negotiation and compromise — techniques that would be adopted decades later by the proponents of the National Health Service.

The act passed by Parliament in 1911 bore little resemblance to Lloyd George's original plan. In 1908, he had met with friendly society representatives who bitterly resented a possible government intrusion into their field. Lloyd George assured the group that he intended to work through the friendly societies and not to destroy them. The resulting compromise led to the creation of "Approved Societies" to administer the national insurance scheme. Another revision was necessary to mollify the insurance industry. This was the abandonment of death benefits. Burial policies were a big money-maker for the insurance organizations, and death benefits threatened to substantially reduce demand for these policies. Other concessions stilled the potential opposition of the doctors. The state had long been employing doctors — as workhouse medical officers, as District Medical Officers providing domiciliary care to the destitute sick, and as public vaccinators. These medical officers generally received low pay, since positions were only filled with those applicants who quoted the lowest acceptable salary. Conditions of practice also proved a source of discontent. Fee-for-service practice, such as exists in the U.S. today, was very limited. Those who could afford to pay for their own medical treatment often joined "medical clubs," where members could contract for care by paying a fixed fee, called a *capitation* fee. Moreover, because it was relatively easy for consumers to compare the fees offered by different contracts, stiff competition kept such fees relatively low.[14]

In general, then, doctors' incomes were relatively modest, and many members of the medical profession were in the mood for a change. The British Medical Association (B.M.A.), as early as 1905, had even proposed the formation of a Public Medical Service by the profession itself. The medical profession, however, almost unanimously opposed Lloyd George's original plan. The opposition centered on two key provisions. First, the plan placed the friendly societies in complete charge of administering the program. In past dealings with the friendly societies, doctors had often felt manipulated by the organizations with which they contracted. They could be dismissed at any time, for any reason, and had no right of appeal. And they were often pressured to sign sickness certificates and insurance forms against their better medical judgment.[15] Thus, doctors feared that under the Lloyd George program their fees would continue to be unacceptably low, and that there would be little improvement in their contractual relations with the friendly societies.

Another concern was the income level below which workers would be compelled to participate, and above which they would be free to refuse participation. Doctors feared that if this income level were set too high, they would lose some of the more lucrative fees they had been able to collect from middle-income patients — fees that were higher than the fees they expected to collect under national health insurance.[16] To demonstrate their opposition, seventy percent of B.M.A. members signed a declaration of non-cooperation in which they pledged not to participate in the scheme.[17] Faced with the threat of such a large doctor boycott, the government raised the minimum capitation fee promised to doctors under the plan. The B.M.A., somewhat mollified, consequently abandoned its opposition to the scheme.

Prelude to the National Health Service

By 1947 some 23 million people — over half the population in Britain over the age of 14 — were covered by national health insurance for medical benefits.[18] The indigent, who were generally not covered by national health insurance, continued to rely on poor-law relief. Moreover, the services of hospitals, which were not covered under the Lloyd George scheme, were becoming increasingly available to the working class through a booming market in private hospital insurance.[19] Nonetheless, all was not well in the British health care market.

One source of complaint was the doctors participating in the national health insurance plan. Between 1913 and 1945, the standard fee paid to a doctor for attending each patient on his "panel" increased by 50 percent. Over the same time period, the average number of physician visits per patient per year also increased by 50 percent (from two visits per year to three visits per year). So the average doctor was doing about 50 percent more work for 50 percent more pay. Yet from 1913 to 1945, consumer prices increased by more than 100 percent.[20]

Doctors also complained about the fact that they had little incentive to maintain the quality of their services under the plan. In general, doctors were paid the same fee regardless of what service was performed. So each doctor had an incentive to provide the bare minimum of service to his patients. They also had an incentive to shuttle their patients off to the hospital sector whenever possible, and to expand the number of patients on their panel in order to increase their total income. Moreover, since medical treatment was "free" to the patients at the time it was received, each patient had an incentive to place exorbitant demands on his doctor. These demands included excessive numbers of prescriptions and requests for sickness certificates which entitled the patient to cash sickness benefits. One investigation into the conditions of general practice summarized its findings this way:

> Excessive numbers of panel patients, and excessive demands for certificates and returns, quickly reduce the general practitioner to an agent for making out prescriptions and for operating something more like a sickness licensing and registration service.[21]

A more widespread complaint, however, stemmed from perceived inequalities that persisted under national health insurance. Since insurance was organized through approved societies, and since these approved societies could select their membership, some inevitably provided better services than others. For example, by carefully screening out the "bad risks," some societies could offer a better deal to its members than others in return for the weekly "premiums." Those groups composed of "good risks" could offer more services, including dental, ophthalmic and even hospital care. Those groups primarily composed of "bad risks" not only offered the bare minimum of services, but many of them were also nearing bankruptcy. The system, therefore, tended to ensure that those workers with the greatest health needs were participating in insurance groups offering the smallest range of medical benefits.[22]

Another source of inequality arose from the distinction between "panel" patients and "private" patients. A common belief was that panel patients received medical care which was inferior to the care received by those who paid directly for medical treatment themselves. This perception was in no way diminished by a political reorganization which consolidated national health insurance and poor-law services under the same ministry.[23]

In the 1920s and 1930s there were numerous recommendations to alter the national health insurance scheme. They included recommendations to extend benefits to the dependents of the insured workers, and to expand the system to cover hospital treatment and other specialist care. Ultimately, these proposals were rejected in favor of a full-fledged, universal scheme of "free" medical care. Many people saw reform of national health insurance as patchwork on a scheme that was fatally flawed in any event. Health care, they argued, should be available to *everyone* as a matter of "right."

But the real reasons why these reforms were rejected were probably political. Initially, the state's contribution to national health insurance had been set at eight percent of the program's total cost. But this contribution soon rose to 25 percent — not an insignificant burden for taxpayers to carry.[24] To have extended coverage, or to have expanded benefits, would have forced politicians to confront some unpalatable options: higher taxes would have had to be imposed on the beneficiaries of the scheme or on the rest of the population.

It seems unlikely that the working class would have been willing to foot a higher tax bill. After all, as individuals they had always retained the option of purchasing wider coverage or expanded benefits through the private insurance market. There would be no political advantage in eliminating this option, unless they could again be convinced that the state was offering "something for nothing." The other alternative seemed equally unpopular. The middle class was already footing a good portion of the bill for national health insurance and receiving no benefit in return. There was little reason to suppose that they wanted to contribute even more.

To the contrary; middle class attitudes were undergoing a profound change. Far from any desire to put more of their tax dollars into working class health benefits, they were becoming of opposite mind — ready to hop on the gravy train themselves. Colm Brogan explains the shift in attitude this way:

[a] large majority of the middle class wanted the Health Service and were determined to get it. The middle-class demand was of profound sociological interest. It had long been the mark of middle-class status to reject welfare benefits. It was unthinkable to live in a subsidized council house. Children had to be educated in private schools, at least in the primary stage, whatever the cost in domestic hardship might be. There were many who thought it demeaning to make use of a free municipal library. These attitudes persist, but only a small minority took the same attitude toward the Health Service. Conscious that they were paying more per head than the working class for benefits which the working class enjoyed almost exclusively, they welcomed the opportunity for getting something, at long last, for their money.[25]

Brogan's observations are profoundly important to an understanding of what the National Health Service is all about today. Early proponents and later defenders of the N.H.S. often described it as a program for redistributing wealth from the middle class to the poor, and for upgrading the quality of health care received by low-income groups to the level enjoyed by the middle class. But this was clearly not the objective of middle-class voters who supported the program. Nor, as we shall see, is it the way the N.H.S. is actually run today.

The National Health Service White Paper, 1944

As early as 1926, there were calls for a unified health service divorced from the insurance system and supported by public funds. Surprisingly, one of the early advocates of such a change was the British Medical Association. In 1942, the B.M.A. published an interim report which called for nothing less than a centrally planned public medical service under government control.[26]

That same year, Sir William Beveridge, architect of the modern British welfare state, issued his famous Beveridge Report. Among other things, the report supported "comprehensive health and rehabilitation services for prevention and cure of disease and restoration of capacity for work, available to all members of the community."[27] The following year, Winston Churchill announced in a national broadcast, "you must rank me and my colleagues as strong partisans of national compulsory insurance for all classes, for all purposes, from cradle to the grave."[28]

In 1944, a White Paper issued by a Coalition Government

(Conservatives, Liberals and Labour) startled no one when it announced:

> The Government believes that, at this stage of social development, the care of personal health should be put on a new footing and be made available to everybody as a publicly sponsored service. Just as people are accustomed to look to public organization for essential facilities like a clean and safe water supply . . . so they should now be able to look for proper facilities for the care of their personal health to a publicly organized service available to all who want to use it.[29]

The plan called for compulsory health "insurance" for the entire population. All medical services were to be made available without charge to the user. Doctors were to be salaried employees of the state. All hospitals were to be nationalized and placed under government control. Private practice, however, was still to be permitted.

Table 2-1 shows what British doctors at the time thought about the White Paper proposal in general, and about a number of specific issues as well. As the table indicates, most of the doctors were opposed to the White Paper. But their objections were to the particulars of the proposal, not to the overall concept. Sixty percent of those responding said they were in favor of a comprehensive system of "free" medical care. Only 37 percent were opposed.

The National Health Service Act, 1946

The victory of the Labour party in 1945, and the arrival of Aneurin Bevan as Minister of Health, worried the B.M.A. — and with good reason. The majority of the medical profession was not adverse to a state-run health service. Many doctors saw it as an opportunity for obtaining better conditions of practice. But one overwhelming fear prevented them from whole-heartedly accepting the N.H.S. — excessive government control, and the resulting loss of clinical and economic freedom. The B.M.A. voiced little opposition to the administrative provisions of the 1946 Act, but its attitude toward Bevan was one of distrust. That attitude was fully vindicated when Bevan refused to negotiate the terms of the Act with the medical profession. Claiming that Parliament was the sovereign body, he insisted that while the doctors could be "consulted," there was no question of negotiation.[30]

To preserve their clinical and economic freedom, the doctors sought the status of "independent contractors" rather than employees

Table 2-1

SELECTED QUESTIONS FROM THE B.M.A. QUESTIONAIRE ON THE WHITE PAPER
(IN PERCENTAGES)

Questions	All		Doctors in Armed Forces		Consultants		G.P.s		Salaried Doctors	
	Pro	Con	Pro	Con	Pro	Con	Pro	Con	Pro	Con
For or against White Paper	39	53	53	41	36	58	31	62	60	33
A 100% service (free comprehensive)	60	37	73	26	54	44	54	43	74	23
Free and complete hospital service	69	28	79	19	58	40	66	32	84	15
Central Administration by Ministry	35	51	45	41	30	57	29	57	49	39
Larger areas for hospital administration	63	24	67	23	64	27	58	26	74	17
"Joint Authorities" for hospital administration	13	78	13	81	9	84	11	79	24	69
Remuneration of consultants by local authorities	37	40	40	40	50	34	30	41	30	44
Central Medical Board for G.P. services	55	31	62	25	50	31	54	35	64	21
Control over G.P.s distribution	57	39	68	28	56	38	51	45	71	25
Health Centers	68	24	83	13	67	23	60	32	83	11
Health Centers practitioners under contract to local authorities	31	53	35	50	29	48	23	63	45	39
Salaried service in Health Centers: full or part time	62	29	74	20	73	25	53	38	79	22
Abolition of sale of practices	56	33	60	28	57	29	53	39	66	19

Source: H. Eckstein, *The English Health Service* (Cambridge, Mass.: Harvard University Press, 1970), Table 3, p. 148. Reprinted by permission.

of the state. In addition, the B.M.A. wanted to restrict coverage under the N.H.S. to only 90 percent of the population. The wealthiest 10 percent of the population, the B.M.A. reasoned, would probably spend more on medical care than the state would spend on their behalf. More importantly, this provision would have ensured that a significant amount of doctors' salaries did not come from the state, thus preventing a complete government monopoly in the employment of medical practitioners. Failing on the 90 percent proposal, the B.M.A. made another one: patients opting for private care should be given a rebate on their contribution to the Health Service. When the government refused to go along with this proposal either, the B.M.A. stiffened its opposition to salaried service — even a partial one.

Using many of the political skills that Lloyd George had mobilized decades earlier, Aneurin Bevan acted quickly to blunt the opposition. His principal tactic: divide and conquer. For example, the hospital consultants (specialists) felt far less threatened by salaried employment than the general practitioners did. By and large, these doctors looked forward to getting paid for hospital work which they had previously performed in an honorary capacity. The consultants were far more concerned with their lucrative private practices.

Bevan allayed their fears with two promises. First, he agreed to allow hospital consultants to accept part-time positions in which they could continue their private practices along with their N.H.S. work. Second, Bevan agreed to set aside a small number of beds in N.H.S. hospitals for private patients. These beds, called "pay beds," would allow consultants to treat their private patients in the same state-owned hospitals where N.H.S. patients were to be treated. One observer described this skillful maneuvering in the following way: "The deal done by Aneurin Bevan with the medical profession in 1946-48 was a simple matter of politics — he bought out the consultants who mattered and ignored the general practitioners and others who did not."[31]

Bevan also offered two plums to the general practioners. First, he agreed to allow G.P.s to practice as independent contractors. Instead of salaried employment, they would receive a fixed (capitation) fee for each patient on their list of patients under the Health Service. Second, he agreed to set aside a certain sum to compensate them for the value of their practice on their retirement (the act forbade the popular technique of "selling" a practice to another G.P.). These concessions were minor, however, compared to those made to the consultants.[32]

Bevan's horsetrading paid off. A poll of doctors in March, 1948, had revealed that 40,814 disapproved of the N.H.S. Act, while only 4,735 expressed approval. Moreover, 25,340 said they were unwilling to serve under the Act.[33] But by the time of a second plebiscite in April, the consultants had left the general practitioners to stand on their own. In advance of the April poll, the B.M.A. announced that if 13,000 of the country's G.P.s voted to refuse service under the N.H.S., the B.M.A. would back a general boycott. Of the 16,129 who voted, 8,493 favored the boycott while 7,636 favored entry into the Health Service. The B.M.A. reluctantly recommended that its members accept service in the N.H.S.[34]

Although over half of the general practitioners had voted to boycott the scheme, the new National Health Service went into operation on the "appointed day," July 5, 1948. Bevan sent a message of goodwill to the doctors:

> There is no reason why the doctor-patient relationship should not be freed from the money factor, the collection of fees or thinking how to pay fees . . . My job is to give you all the facilities, resources, apparatus and help I can, and then to leave you alone . . . to use your skill and judgment without hindrance.[35]

Over thirty years later, as we shall see, doctors have discovered a great many reasons why the doctor-patient relationship should not be "freed from the money factor."

Footnotes

1. Dennis Lees, "Economics and Non-economics of Health Services," *Three Banks Review*, 110, June, 1976, p. 11.
2. Economic Models, Ltd., *The British Health Care System* (Chicago: American Medical Association, 1976), p. 16.
3. *Ibid*, p. 16.
4. Maurice Bruce, *The Coming of the Welfare State* (London: B.T. Batsford Ltd., 1966) p. 37. Concern over taxes, according to Bruce, "could even attain, however logically, the depths of the ludicrous. A case is recorded in which it was solemnly argued before the Justices which of two parishes was liable for a pauper whose house, and even whose bed, stood on the actual parish boundary — the decision being that the settlement went with the man's head as he lay in bed!"
5. Bruce, *The Coming of the Welfare State*, p. 103.
6. Economic Models, Ltd., *The British Health Care System*, p. 16.
7. Mathew J. Lynch and Stanley S. Raphael, *Medicine and the State* (Oak Brook, Illinois: Association of American Physicians and Surgeons, 1973), p. 117.
8. Bentley B. Gilbert, *The Evolution of National Insurance in Great Britain* (London: Michael Joseph Ltd., 1966), p. 167.
9. See Gilbert, *The Evolution of National Insurance*, chapters 4 and 6, for a thorough discussion of the friendly societies and their political influence.
10. Economic Models, Ltd., *The British Health Care System*, p. 22.
11. Colm Brogan, "Shortages as Seen by a Journalist," in Helmut Schoeck, ed., *Financing Medical Care* (Caldwell, Idaho: Caxton Printers, Ltd., 1962), p. 54.
12. Sidney and Beatrice Webb were prominent leaders in the Fabian Socialist movement around the turn of the century.
13. Brogan, "Shortages as Seen by a Journalist," p. 13.
14. Economic Models, Ltd., *The British Health Care System*, p. 22.
15. *Ibid*.
16. Lynch and Raphael, *Medicine and the State*, p. 123.
17. Economic Models, Ltd., *The British Health Care System*, p. 23.
18. Lynch and Raphael, *Medicine and the State*, p. 124.
19. Economic Models, Ltd., *The British Health Care System*, pp. 26-27.
20. Lynch and Raphael, *Medicine and the State*, p. 125.
21. *Ibid*.
22. Economic Models, Ltd., *The British Health Care System*, p. 28.
23. Bruce, *The Coming of the Welfare State*, p. 211.
24. Lynch and Raphael, *Medicine and the State*, p. 125.
25. Brogan, "Shortages As Seen by a Journalist," p. 57.
26. Economic Models, Ltd., *The British Health Care System*, pp. 29-30.
27. Sir William Beveridge, *Social Insurance and Allied Services* (New York: The Macmillan Company, 1942), p. 120.
28. Quoted in Lynch and Raphael, *Medicine and the State*, p. 136.
29. Bruce, *The Coming of the Welfare State*, p. 259.
30. Economic Models, Ltd., *The British Health Care System*, p. 68.
31. Lees, "Economics and Non-economics of Health Services," pp. 11-12.
32. Economic Models, Ltd., *The British Health Care System*, pp. 69-70.
33. Lynch and Raphael, *Medicine and the State*, pp. 142-143.
34. *Ibid*, pp. 144-145.
35. Bruce, *The Coming of the Welfare State*. p. 284.

Chapter 3
The Organization of British Health Care Today

All residents of (and most visitors to) Britain today are eligible for a wide range of health care services. These include the services of physicians and hospitals, laboratory tests, dental and ophthalmic care and drug prescriptions. They also include a great many services that U.S. citizens do not normally expect — house calls by general practitioners, home nurses and health visitors and a vast array of personal services for the elderly, the chronically ill and the handicapped.

Virtually all of these services are free of cost to the patient at time of treatment. In the few exceptions (introduced since 1948) to this rule, the charges are usually nominal. For example, patients pay about 40 cents for most drug prescriptions and about eight dollars for eye glasses.[1] Moreover, most of these charges are waived for low-income groups, the elderly and children. There are no charges for basic medical care — the medical services of physicians and hospitals.

Although all British citizens are eligible for "free" medical care, they do not necessarily receive all of the medical care that they want, or even all of the care that doctors decide that they need. One of the ironies of the British health care system is that the system was originally proposed, and subsequently defended, on the theory that health care should be made available as a matter of "right" and not on the basis of ability to pay. In fact, however, Parliament has never granted individuals the "right" to any specific course of treatment for any specific illness.[2] And the abridgement of the theoretical "right" to health care, as we shall see, is a daily routine in Britain, especially in the hospital sector.

This is one of the reasons why health care provided on the basis of ability to pay has never vanished in Britain. Individuals may contract privately with general practitioners, specialists and private hospitals and nursing homes. A small percentage of beds in state-owned hospitals is also reserved for private care. Moreover, as in the United States, in the private British health care market people may have access to all the care for which they (or their insurance companies) are willing to pay.

State financed health care services are, of course, not really "free." Ultimately, these services are paid for through direct and indirect taxes on the patients who use the services. As Table 3-1 shows, the lion's share of spending by National Health Service is financed through general taxes collected at the national and local level. Slightly less than five percent is financed through the social security payroll tax ("N.H.S. contribution"), and another four percent comes from the small number of user fees.

Table 3-1

SPENDING AND SOURCES OF FINANCE FOR THE NATIONAL HEALTH SERVICE

England, 1975/76

SPENDING

	£ million	%
Health Authorities: Current Expenditure	3,129	57.9
Health Authorities: Capital Expenditure	332	6.1
Personal Social Services	869	16.1
Pharmaceutical Services	390	7.2
General Medical Services	280	5.2
General Dental Services	201	3.7
General Ophthalmic Services	62	1.2
Central Administration	34	0.6
Welfare Foods	13	0.2
Other	96	1.8
	5,406	100.0

SOURCES OF FINANCE

	£ million	%
General Taxes (excluding grants to local authorities)	4,030	74.5
Local Taxes and Consolidated Fund grants	777	14.4
N.H.S. Contribution	398	7.4
Payment by Users	187	3.5
Other	14	0.2
	5,406	100.0

Source: Department of Health and Social Security, *Health and Personal Social Services Statistics for England* (London: Her Majesty's Stationery Office, 1977), Tables 2.4 and 2.5, pp. 20-21.

Administrative Structure

The structure chosen for the N.H.S. in 1948 reflected Bevan's desire to accommodate various factions in the medical profession far more than it reflected a desire for an efficiently managed health care system. The general practitioners, dentists, opticians and pharmacists wanted the status of "independent contractors" rather than that of salaried employees. They also wanted to be free of the administrative power of local governments. Hospital doctors and administrators were equally fearful of the power of local governments, and sought to maintain their independence from other sectors of the N.H.S. as well.

The upshot of these negotiations was the tripartite structure illustrated in Figure 3-1. Both the hospital sector and the primary medical sector were established as independent branches of the N.H.S. Each had its own administrative hierarchy leading directly to the Secretary of State in the Department of Health and Social Security (D.H.S.S.). The local authorities were left in charge of such services as home nursing, ambulance service, community health centers, etc. Note the special line of authority granted to the hospital consultants.

Figure 3-1

Administrative Structure of the National Health Service in England & Wales
1948-1974

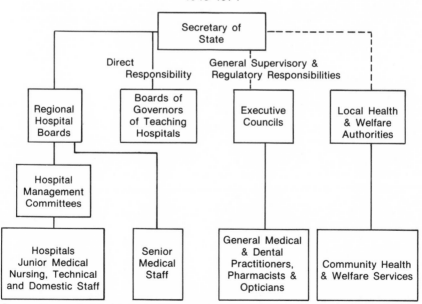

Source: Economic Models Ltd., *The British Health Care System* (Chicago: American Medical Association, 1976), p. 38. Reprinted with the permission of the American Medical Association.

One of the great disadvantages of the structure shown in Figure 3-1 is that there is no mechanism for coordinating the activities of the three sectors except at the top of the organizational chart. By 1974, administrative inefficiencies in the N.H.S. had become so glaring that a complete reorganization of the health service was made.[3]

The 1974 reorganization established a four-tier system of control. Under the D.H.S.S. level, there are now 14 Regional Health Authorities, 90 Area Health Authorities, and 206 Districts. In addition there are about 207 Community Health Councils representing the views of health consumers, and a myriad of "gap-bridging" committees and less formal organizations. Figure 3-2 depicts the British government's view of how the new organization works.

As one might expect, soon after the reorganization took place the terms "red tape" and "cumbersome bureaucracy" were heard more and more frequently both inside and outside the N.H.S. Many began to wonder whether the four-tier system represented any improvement over the old system. As one health official put it, "Everyone agrees that it would be nice to eliminate at least one tier; the only one viewed as dispensable by officials outside of London, however, is the D.H.S.S. itself."[4]

The Budgetary Costs of the NHS

Given the inordinate amount of attention devoted to health care costs in the United States in recent years, a natural question to ask about the British system is: *how has the system performed in holding down health care costs?* The question sounds reasonable. But, in fact, it is not a particularly meaningful question.

One way to keep the national health bill down is simply to spend less. This is particularly easy to do in a country like Britain, where 95 percent of all spending on health care is done by the government. In theory, the British government could reduce its health bill to zero by choosing to spend nothing at all. Of course if the British government chose not to purchase any health care services, then none would be provided — at least not to N.H.S. patients.

But this is not what most people have in mind when they ask about health care costs. Everyone realizes that our health bill could be lowered by choosing to purchase fewer health services. What interests most people in the United States is not whether we can reduce the amount of health care we consume, but whether we can have the same health services we now have for a lower price. Have the British

Figure 3-2

ORGANIZATIONAL STRUCTURE OF NHS

Source: Department of Health and Social Security.

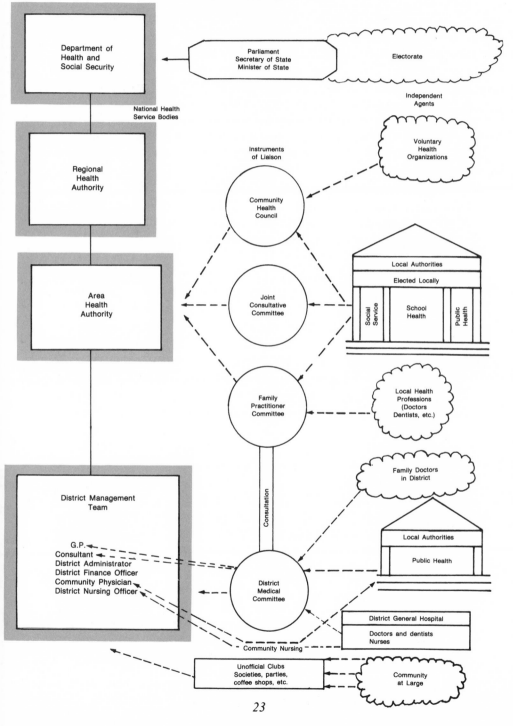

succeeded in keeping the price of health services lower than comparable services in America?

The answer, I believe, is clearly *no*. But this is not an answer that is easy to substantiate with numbers. For one thing, British patients do not generally receive the same health services that American patients receive. The average British citizen consumes less health care than his American counterpart, and the health care that is consumed in Britain is of a lower quality. For another, in order to receive health care in Britain, patients must bear a great many personal, non-monetary costs that American patients do not experience. These are personal costs that are difficult to calculate in terms of dollars and cents.

Most Americans have a vague impression that health care costs have soared under the British system of socialized medicine. In terms of nominal spending, the impression is correct. Within eight months of the beginning of the N.H.S., government officials discovered that they had underestimated the N.H.S. budget by one-third.[5] The total N.H.S. budget tripled in ten years.[6] But these figures are misleading.

Compared to other countries in the world, Britain's health care budget can be described as stingy. As Table 3-2 shows, Britain spends only about one-third as much per person on health services as the United States. In fact, per capita spending on health care in Britain is lower than in just about any major industrialized country.

Another way to look at spending on health care is to compare total medical expenditure to gross national product. In most countries, as citizens become wealthier they devote a larger fraction of their income to medical care. Worldwide, there is a clear, positive relationship between gross national product per capita and the fraction of GNP devoted to health care.[7] But as Figure 3-3 shows, during the early years of the N.H.S., the British trend was in the opposite direction. In fact, the British were spending the same percent of GNP on health care in 1965 as they were 15 years earlier. In recent years, however, the fraction of GNP devoted to health care has been rising. But as Table 3-2 shows, by this measure, Britain's spending on health care still ranks among the lowest in the industrialized world.

Commenting on statistics like these, Dennis Lees, Professor of Economics at the University of Nottingham, recently wrote:

Contrary to popular belief, especially abroad, the British N.H.S. has not been costly but disastrously cheap. It has had constantly low political priority in public expenditure and, as

Table 3-2

TOTAL MEDICAL CARE EXPENDITURE PER CAPITA AND AS A
PERCENTAGE OF "TREND" GROSS DOMESTIC PRODUCT[1]
(1976 or near date)

COUNTRY	MEDICAL CARE EXPENDITURE PER CAPITA (in 1976 US dollars)	MEDICAL CARE EXPENDITURE: PERCENTAGE OF TREND GDP	
Australia	$427	6.5%	(1975/76)
Austria	333	5.7	
Canada	548	6.8	(1973)
Finland	383	5.8	(1975)
France	531	6.9	
Germany	645	6.7	
Italy	190	6.0	
Netherlands	566	7.3	
Norway	500	5.6	(1973)
Sweden	793	7.3	
United Kingdom	188	5.2	(1975)
United States	593	7.4	

1. "Trend" Gross Domestic Product is used in place of actual GDP in order to avoid the potentially distorting effects of cyclical economic fluctuation.

Source: For estimates of per capita expenditure, data on total health spending is taken from *World Health Spending Outlook to 1990,* No. 157 (Cleveland, Ohio: Predicast, Inc., 1979). Population statistics are estimated as of July 1, 1975, and are taken from Population Reference Bureau, *World Population Growth and Response: 1965-1975* (Washington, D.C., April, 1976), pp. 267-271. Data on health expenditure as a percent of GDP is taken from Organization for Economic Co-operation and Development, *Public Expenditure on Health* (Paris: OECD, 1977), Table 1, p. 10.

a proportion of national income, is one of the lowest among industrial countries. So there has not been more medical care as a result of nationalization and tax finance. In fact, the British people, left free to do so, would almost certainly have chosen to spend more on health services themselves than governments have chosen to spend on their behalf.[8]

Why "disastrously cheap"? Because part of the price the British pay for so little N.H.S. spending is that they are often denied medical care that doctors admit they need. Those who receive medical care often do so at considerable cost — including months, and even years, of waiting while living in pain. Today there are over 750,000 waiting to enter British hospitals.[9]

American health expert Harry Swartz summarized conditions in

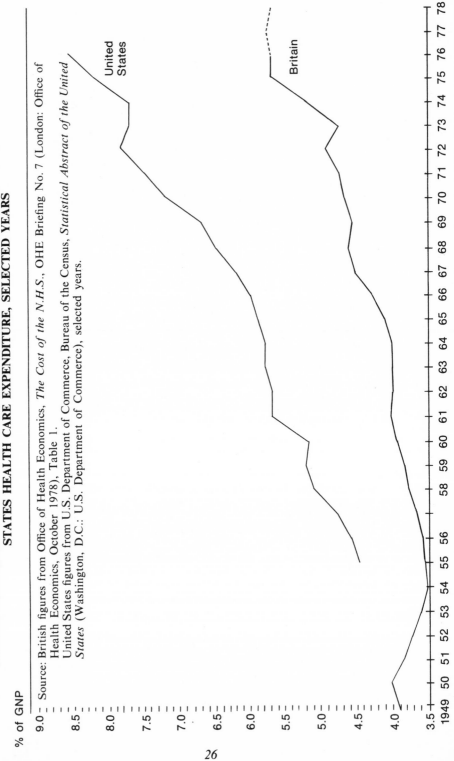

Figure 3-3

HEALTH CARE EXPENDITURE AS A PERCENTAGE OF GNP UNITED KINGDOM, 1949-1978. UNITED STATES HEALTH CARE EXPENDITURE, SELECTED YEARS

Source: British figures from Office of Health Economics, *The Cost of the N.H.S.*, OHE Briefing No. 7 (London: Office of Health Economics, October 1978), Table 1.
United States figures from U.S. Department of Commerce, Bureau of the Census, *Statistical Abstract of the United States* (Washington, D.C.: U.S. Department of Commerce), selected years.

this way: "The fact is that by American standards, the N.H.S. is a meager and Spartan medical system, many of whose economics would be regarded as inhuman brutality if applied to Americans."[10] In the following chapters we will look at some examples of this "brutality," as well as a great many other "costs" that British patients must bear. Before we do that, however, we need to take a close look at some general principles of health economics.

Footnotes

1. Mary-Ann Rozbicki, *Rationing British Health Care: The Cost/Benefit Approach.* Executive Seminar in National and International Affairs (Washington, DC: U.S. Department of State, 1977), p. 4.
2. Rudolf Klein, "British Doctors Must Decide Whom to Save," *Chicago Tribune,* September 6, 1978. (Rudolf Klein is Professor of Social Policy Studies at the University of Bath, England.)
3. Economic Models, Ltd., *The British Health Care System* (Chicago: American Medical Association, 1976), p. 41.
4. Quoted in Rozbicki, *Rationing British Health Care,* p. 3.
5. Mathew Lynch and Stanley Raphael, *Medicine and the State* (Oak Brook, Illinois: Association of American Physicians and Surgeons, 1973), p. 178-179.
6. Stuart Butler and Eamonn Butler, *The British National Health Service in Theory and Practice* (Washington, D.C.: The Heritage Foundation, 1974), p. 4.
7. See, for example, Joseph P. Newhouse and George A. Goldberg, *Allocation of Resources in Medical Care From an Economic Viewpoint: Remarks to the XXIX World Assembly of the World Medical Assocation and Commentary* (Santa Monica, California: The Rand Corporation, 1976), pp. 6-9.
8. Dennis Lees, "Economics and Non-economics of Health Services," *Three Banks Review,* 110, June, 1976, p. 9.
9. Jonathan Spivak, "Private Health Care in Britain," *Wall Street Journal,* August 21, 1979.
10. Harry Swartz, "The Infirmity of British Medicine," in R. Emmett Tyrrell, Jr., ed., *The Future that Doesn't Work: Social Democracy's Failures in Britain* (Garden City, New York: Doubleday, 1977), p. 30.

Chapter 4
The National Health Service and Some General Principles of Health Economics

For many American automobile owners, the winter of 1973-74 jostles some bitter memories. That was the winter when an Arab oil embargo caused a sharp cutback in gasoline available to motorists. Because there was less gasoline to be consumed, motorists could not purchase as much as they had become accustomed to purchasing. The process of adjustment was, at best, annoying; at worst, painful. But it was even more distressing for a special reason: government price controls were in force at the time.

Before the embargo, the price of gasoline was about 50 cents per gallon in most parts of the country. At that price, motorists were buying all of the gasoline they wanted to buy. After the embargo, the price remained at 50 cents, but there was a lot less gasoline to go around. That's when motorists discovered they could no longer buy as much gas as they wanted. That's also when chaos set in.

Under ordinary circumstances, the price of gasoline would have jumped to about 85 cents at many service stations. In some parts of the country, the price might well have reached one dollar. Motorists would certainly have been disappointed. But in the face of higher prices, they would have done what consumers always do when the price of something rises — they would have voluntarily reduced the amount of gasoline they purchased. A higher price encourages consumers to conserve. It is one way of rationing a limited quantity of gasoline among the many consumers who would like to have it.

As it turns out, things were quite different after the Arab oil embargo. Since service stations were not allowed to raise their prices, some other method of rationing had to be found. Most rationed their supplies on the basis of first come/first served.

In the more extreme cases, it worked something like this: at selected intervals, a station would receive a new allotment of gasoline from its supplier. As soon as they learned gas was available, car owners quickly responded. Long lines of automobiles formed in front of the station and cars were serviced until the supply was exhausted. In New York City and some metropolitan areas of New Jersey, drivers would typically wait two or three hours before they could reach an available pump. Even then there was no assurance that gas would be available by the time their turn arrived.

For some drivers, the wait was considerably longer. News that a depleted station was about to receive a new supply of gas could lead to the formation of lines of cars up to a half-day in advance. Lines would sometimes form on the basis of rumors. A few hardy souls even parked their cars in front of service stations overnight.

For many consumers, the result was somewhat shocking. The idea of holding the price of gasoline to 50 cents initially had widespread approval. But motorists soon learned that even though the price at the pump was only 50 cents, the "price" they actually had to pay was far more than 50 cents. The real price was 50 cents in the form of money *plus* several hours of wasted time.

Some people missed work, which often meant a loss of salary. Other people gave up valuable leisure time. All had one thing in common—in order to buy gasoline, they had to wait, wait, wait![1]

Naturally a lot of clever motorists tried to find ways to avoid the long waits — and there were ways. The British would call these practices "line jumping" or "queue jumping." During the winter of 1973-74, a shrewd automobile owner could sometimes "beat the system." The local service station attendant could be very appreciative of a gift of a good bottle of scotch or a handsome tip on occasion. Thus, for some the long waits were avoided. But not for everyone.

Waiting was not the only inconvenience most motorists had to suffer. A lot of service stations refused to completely fill a tank when a car reached an available pump. On the theory that as many cars as possible should be serviced, many attendants refused to give motorists more than one-half a tank full, or even one-third.

Service stations also did something else — they reduced the quality of the services they rendered. After all, service stations had no reason to worry about losing customers to a competitor. The line of potential customers extended for blocks. So they neglected to clean windshields, check the pressure in tires, check oil levels and batteries, and perform many of the other services customers had grown to expect.

One other feature of our experiment in rationing gasoline deserves mentioning — politics. During the 1973-74 crisis, government bureaucrats allocated fuel production between gasoline and diesel fuel. In making their decisions, they faced strong political pressures. Truckers claimed they needed more diesel fuel than they were getting, and demanded more. Of course motorists also thought they needed more gasoline. But the independent truckers associations were better organized. They initiated a strike and threatened to paralyze the country unless their demands were met. To ensure "cooperation," they blocked roads, vandalized equipment and generally harassed nonstriking truckers. Eventually the regulators succumbed and raised the production of diesel fuel. This move, however, was later overturned in the courts.

The rationing of gasoline during the mid-1970s among service stations was also a sensitive political issue. Many operators were accused of getting unfair amounts because of political influence. One of those so accused was Billy Carter, brother of U.S. President Jimmy Carter. Carter denied the charge, claiming that he received more gasoline because he needed it. Of course, during the gasoline rationing crisis, everybody "needed" more; and it was never quite clear why some needs were satisfied while others went unmet.

Despite all the problems just described, things could have been much worse. Let's suppose for a moment that, instead of a controlled price of 50 cents per gallon, the government had insisted that gasoline be given away absolutely free. What would have happened?

The waiting lines would have been much longer, and the amount allocated per car much smaller. Deterioration in the quality of service would also have been much greater, line jumping more frequent, and political pressures more severe. In short, whatever chaos we endured with gasoline rationing was minor compared to how bad it *could* have been.

So what does all this have to do with health care? A great deal. Instead of giving gasoline to consumers for "free," the British government makes health care available to consumers with virtually no charge to the user. What's more, every problem we encountered with gasoline rationing in the United States has a parallel in the British health care market.

Take waiting, for example. British patients wait and wait and wait. They wait to get an appointment with their doctors. They wait in doctors' offices. After being referred to a specialist, they wait again for an appointment. On the day of their appointment, they wait even more. And, if they get the OK for any serious medical treatment, the waiting *really* begins. Patients who are scheduled for operations, for example, can end up waiting for years.

As in the case of gasoline rationing, British doctors are faced with the problem of allocating their limited time among the increasing demands placed upon them. One way they do this is by spending less, and less time with each patient. Whereas American doctors spend an average of about 15 minutes with each patient, in Britain the average time spent is less than five minutes. The average British patient, in other words, gets about one-third of a tank full.

Moreover, just as service station attendants eliminated a great many services to their customers, so British doctors have eliminated a great many services that American patients expect as a matter of course. In the first place, the incentives not to do so are weak. Instead of having cars lined down the block, the typical British doctor has his office jammed full of patients. For most of them, there is little fear of losing customers to a competitor. In the second place, the British doctor simply does not have the time to provide "full service" to all his patients — even if he were so inclined. The upshot is that most British patients miss out on the medical equivalent of having their batteries, oil level and tire pressure checked.

In Britain, too, there is "line jumping." If you're willing to pay more, you can move to the head of the line. But this is a privilege of which only a small minority of patients can take advantage. There are also constant political pressures on the National Health Service to place the needs and interests of some groups ahead of others. All too frequently, entire hospitals have been closed because of strikes by hospital personnel.

On top of this, British health care has one crucial feature that was missing from our experiment in gasoline rationing: in Britain, the suppliers of medical services are paid by the government. Under gasoline rationing, service stations in the United States still operate as private businesses. For this reason, the station owners had a large incentive to keep costs down by running an efficient operation. Were the stations owned and operated by the government, they no doubt would have been far less efficient.

In fact, in order to complete our analogy, one has to perform the following thought experiment: think back to the days when gasoline was rationed by waiting. Try to imagine what the situation would have been like were the prices lowered from 50 cents per gallon to zero. Also try to imagine service stations managed and operated by a large governmental organization like the U.S. Postal Service. If your imagination can stretch that far, then you have an excellent mental picture of a system which is quite comparable to the British National Health Service.

Is Health Care Different?

Some readers may reasonably question whether health care and gasoline are really comparable. Aren't these products quite different? If they are different, isn't an analogy between the two very misleading? It turns out that there *are* differences between the two products, and these differences do make the analogy slightly misleading. But the dissimilarities and the difference they make may surprise you. Actually, the problems we confronted in the gasoline market tend to understate the problems that arise when medical care is rationed. In the market for medical care, the chaos that results is much worse!

Every student who takes a course in economics comes face to face with the most important principle that discipline has to offer — *the law of demand*. The principle is really quite simple. It says that the quantity that consumers will be willing to buy of a good or service will rise if the price is lowered. We are discouraged by high prices and encouraged by low ones.

Most students introspect and agree that the principle is indeed a reasonable one. They can think of all kinds of products they might be purchasing if only the price were lower. It's not difficult to see why people would buy less gasoline when the price is high and more gasoline when the price is low. The same principle surely applies to automobiles, television sets, and just about every other product we can think of.

But what about health care? Does the principle really apply here? From the very day when the first economist sat down to apply the tools of his trade to this field, he began to ask himself if the tools were really applicable. Is health care different?

At first glance, some students may conclude that it *is* different. After all, they reason, "When I am sick, I go to the doctor. When I am not sick, I do not go to the doctor. It's as simple as that. Prices, and in particular doctors' fees, have nothing whatever to do with my decision."

My response to statements like this is to ask my students to introspect again. Isn't it true, I query, that you do not always see a doctor when you are sick? Isn't it also true, I ask, that in making the decision to see a doctor you consciously, or unconsciously, consider the "costs" of doing so, including travel time, waiting time, and other inconveniences? If a doctor were living in your household and you could consult him at virtually zero costs, wouldn't you consult him more often than you consult your actual doctor? In reflecting on these questions, students gradually begin to realize something about their own behavior and the behavior of other people as well — *the law of demand applies to health care too.*

Not only can this truth be grasped by honest introspection, it has been confirmed repeatedly by virtually every economic study in the field of health care.[2] The demand for the services of general practitioners, the demand for hospital services — indeed, the demand for virtually every medical service — varies inversely with the price charged to the user.

Most of the economic studies of the demand for health care have been conducted in the United States and Canada. But there is considerable evidence that the same principle holds true for the British system as well. This can be seen by observing how demand responds to price changes in one of the few areas of the N.H.S. where a fee is imposed — prescription drugs. In the early days of the N.H.S., prescription drugs were made free to the user. But when the use of these drugs subsequently soared, the N.H.S. faced severe financial strains in meeting its annual pharmaceutical bill.

Among those who did not care to inquire into the economic basis for this phenomenon, there were frequent charges that the drug companies were "profiteers in sickness" and that the British people were "a nation of hypochondriacs."[3] Despite these attacks, an "economic" solution was quickly found. In 1952, the N.H.S. began charging a fee for prescriptions. The fee was raised in 1956 and again in 1961. Each time the fee was raised, the number of prescriptions fell off sharply. But as other prices and incomes rose, the upward trend of prescriptions gradually resumed.

In 1965, the Labour Party abolished prescription charges altogether. The results were dramatic. In three years, the number of prescriptions rose by 30 percent. Charges were reintroduced in 1968, and within two years, the number of prescriptions fell by 10 percent.[4]

Two other areas in the N.H.S. where fees were charged — dentistry and ophthamology — also offer powerful testimony to the importance of the law of demand. In 1951, the N.H.S. began charging patients for about one-half the cost of dentures. Over the following year, the number of dentures fell by 60 percent. Similarly, when a charge of £1 (plus actual cost of frames) was introduced for spectacles in 1951, the number of spectacles issued also fell by 60 percent.[5]

The recognition that the law of demand applies to health care, and that it is a very important principle underlying the way in which people behave, is sometimes called the *economic approach* to health care. The term is an apt one, for virtually all modern health economists, regardless of their political view, accept its validity.

This approach is a fairly modern one, however, and is by no means accepted by most noneconomists. An important alternative, often advanced by doctors and politicians (including those who established the N.H.S.), is the *technological approach*. This is the approach taken by those who assert that "only sickness matters;" or its corollary, "only sickness *should* matter." Advocates of this approach typically believe that the price of medical care deters very few people, except perhaps the very poor. In any event, they argue, price should not determine the quantity or quality of the medical care people receive. What should? Medical need.

An example of this approach in the United States is an important medical study that was conducted in the 1930's [6] and recently updated in the prestigious *New England Journal of Medicine.* [7] All such studies proceed in a typical fashion — they estimate the total amount of sickness in a given population and then estimate the amount of medical services (physicians, hospitals, etc.) that are "necessary" to treat that amount of sickness. The 1930's study, for example, estimated that 135 physicians would be necessary for every 100,000 people.

This was precisely the approach toward health care taken by the founders of the N.H.S. Aneurin Bevan and William Beveridge, for example, did believe that some British citizens were deterred from seeking medical care by the price of that care. For this reason, they believed that there were medical needs that were going untreated. With medical care free to the user, however, such people would no longer be deterred. As a result, they expected that the N.H.S. would initially be confronted with a backlog of untreated sickness.

Once this backlog had been eliminated, however, Bevan expected health expenditures to stabilize. In fact, he eventually thought health care expenditures would decline. With health care free to the user, more British citizens would avail themselves of preventive care. Preventive care would nip sickness in the bud, so to speak, and thus be an investment which yielded returns in the form of lower health expenditures in future years.

The arguments sounded persuasive at the time. But almost thirty years after the N.H.S. was established, a former Minister of Health declared that the term "medical need" was "meaningless,"[8] and that "there is virtually no limit to the amount of medical care an individual is capable of absorbing."[9] A few years later, a British health economist stated, "We could easily spend the entire GNP of Britain on the health service — and still want more."[10]

At first glance, these comments might appear to be an exaggeration. True, there probably is a definite limit to the number of prescriptions, eyeglasses and dentures the British can absorb. But when all of the services of the N.H.S. are considered, there is no visible limit to the quantity of service the British could consume. Not only could the entire GNP of Britain be spent on health care, the British could probably spend several times that amount — and still want more.

What is true for Britain is also true for the United States. It is for this reason that I confessed that the analogy between gasoline and health care is somewhat misleading. The amount of gasoline that Americans can consume is undoubtedly well below our GNP. After all, there are only so many automobiles and there is only so much driving time. But in the area of health care, the opportunities for potential consumption are almost limitless.

Because this conclusion is at once so surprising, and at the same time so crucial to an understanding of what the market for health care is all about, let's take a closer look at the "need" versus "demand" distinction.

Medical "Need" Versus Medical "Demand"

Where did Aneurin Bevan go wrong? How was it that he so totally misperceived the nature of the market for health care in Britain? Bevan's mistakes were several, and they are shared by practically all those who take the technological approach toward health.

In the first place, Bevan, along with so many others, completely misperceived the nature of "illness." What most health experts realize today is that virtually everyone is to some degree "ill." This realization dawned only gradually, and, in part, came about because of the rather startling results of general surveys of the public health.

An early British survey, conducted in the late 1930's, reported that 26 percent of those questioned claimed to be suffering from one or more forms of illness.[11] A decade later in another public survey, 75 percent of those questioned claimed to have suffered from ill health during the preceding month.[12] In the early 1970's, two more surveys found that 95 percent of those questioned had experienced one or more symptoms of ill health during the fourteen days prior to questioning.[13]

Is the state of British health in rapid decline? There has clearly been a substantial rise in the percentage of the population that think they are sick. One of the problems with these surveys, however, is that they asked people to evaluate their own health. Obviously, different people can have widely different abilities to perform this task.

The 1930's survey confirms this suspicion. In that study, people were actually given a physical examination in addition to being questioned. Although only 26 percent of those examined thought they were ill, the examinations revealed that over 90 percent had some identifiable sickness.

How do these results compare to the state of health in more recent times? In 1968, multiple screening tests were carried out in Southward, England. Out of 1,000 people examined, 93 percent had some identifiable sickness.[14] The examiners, then, found slightly more illness in 1968 than was found in the late 1930's — despite the fact that between the 1930's and 1968 there were enormous advances in medical technology, and considerable expansion in the availability of doctors, hospitals and public health services.

The British government's own national morbidity (sickness) tables show a more dramatic rise in sickness for the population as a whole. Ruth Levitt recently compared British morbidity tables for 1955/56 with those published later, for 1970/71. She found an increase of 36 percent in morbidity between the two surveys.[15]

What happened? It is tempting to conclude that the British are becoming less and less healthy. This conclusion is probably wrong, however. Surveys of public health in practically any country over the past 30 or 40 years would probably show a similar rise in morbidity. Why? Because, as time passes, our ability to diagnose illness improves. And the better our ability to diagnose, the more illness we find!

Modern medical technology not only improves our ability to *cure* illness, it also improves our ability to *find* it. As medical technology becomes even more sophisticated, we will undoubtedly find even more illness. There is no reason whatever to believe that we will ever reach a point when we will cease discovering new and different kinds of illness.

Considerations such as these have given rise to a familiar comment in health economics — the only fit man is one who has been inadequately examined by his doctor. To this we should probably add the following: if an adequate examination pronounces a man fit, it is only because the tools of examination are too primitive.

One way to appreciate this fact is to consider the following hypothesis about illness. Unless we die of accident, suicide, homicide, or the like, each of us will die because something inside us malfunctions. Someday, something inside our bodies will stop working. Since we can predict that this will happen with great confidence, it does not seem unreasonable to suppose that the "seeds" of our demise are germinating in us right now.

If this hypothesis is correct, then we are all certainly "ill". For we contain inside us the potential ultimate causes of our death. Current medical technology does not give us the ability to detect the early "seeds" of cancer, heart attacks, strokes and many other life-threatening conditions. That is, we don't really know why these conditions occur, although we have some limited ability to treat them once they do occur. Of course, some day we may discover that by giving some sort of medical treatment to a child, we may prevent the onset of cancer, stroke or heart disease for the rest of his life. But if that happens, then the child will ultimately die of some other cause and we will have to search for a treatment for *that* illness.

Even if you do not accept the hypothesis that all of us are ill in the conventional sense, it is difficult to deny that most of us are "ill" in an unconventional sense — we age! Some medical researchers actually regard aging as a form of illness. And right now there is research being conducted to find a chemical "cure" for the "disease" of aging.[16]

There are also some other unconventional notions of "illness" in use these days. New and exotic research is being conducted into ways of altering the DNA make-up of our genes. The prospective results are impressive. Scientists expect to be able to prevent genetic defects in children, and even alter their susceptibility to disease.

Is aging really an illness? Is a genetic defect or a genetic susceptibility to disease an illness? One thing is for certain: medical science is rapidly expanding the horizons of what is possible in order to improve our health. It is precisely because these horizons are so broad and so all-encompassing that the former Minister of Health was able to declare "medical need" meaningless. He might have gone on to say that, even if we steadfastly insist on using the term, we are forced to admit that the "need," like the demand, for medical care is infinite.

Bevan's first mistake, then, was to fail to perceive that there is no limit to, and perhaps not even a definition of, what our medical "needs" really are. His second mistake was closely related — he believed there were definite and only moderately expensive methods of treating illness.

The N.H.S. was founded in the days before the pioneering developments in treating illness were discovered. Its founders knew nothing of micro-surgery, open-heart surgery, hip replacements, kidney transplants, and dozens of other medical techniques — all of which could easily bankrupt the N.H.S. and perhaps Britain as well, if used to their full potential.

As an example of the enormous potential for spending money on treatment, consider the CAT scanner. It's a marvelous innovation in medical technology. With it, medical technicians can "see" into the body and detect brain tumors, the presence of heart disease, damage from a heart attack, and a great many other conditions that could previously be analyzed only with surgery.[17]

As they are currently used, CAT scanners are mainly reserved for patients who are thought to be seriously ill. But they also have enormous potential in preventive medicine, something that was near and dear to Bevan's heart. A CAT scanner, for example, can detect lung cancer in very early stages — long before it can be detected by conventional X-ray. It can also detect many other life-threatening conditions in their early stages. As a result, a person who is otherwise quite healthy can benefit from a stint under the scanner in the same way that he can benefit from any other form of medical check-up.

The trouble with CAT scanners is that they are expensive. Some of the latest models cost over $2 million. In addition, they require highly trained technicians to operate them and very skilled medical personnel to interpret the results. As far as I can tell, every British citizen would benefit from an annual scanner check-up. But the total cost of all of those checkups would exceed the entire current budget of the N.H.S.

Bevan's third mistake was the direct consequence of the first two — he failed to perceive that *medical care must be rationed.* On the one hand, as we have seen, the ability of the British to usefully consume medical care is virtually unlimited. On the other hand, the resources available to supply medical care are quite limited. If the British can not satisfy all of their health needs by spending their entire GNP on medical care, it is clear that they will be able to satisfy far fewer needs by spending only six or seven percent of their GNP on medical care. Only a fraction of medical needs, then, can be met. By necessity, the majority of needs must go unmet.

It is interesting to speculate how Bevan might have responded to this problem. Since he wholeheartedly endorsed the technological view of health care, he probably would have preferred a technological answer — the most important needs should receive priority. This is the answer given by a great many doctors and administrators in the N.H.S. It is also the answer recently proposed by Anthony Culyer, a noted British health economist.

Culyer argues that the purpose of the N.H.S. should be to minimize the state of ill health in Britain.[18] He also proposes a rather innovative scheme by which health needs might be ranked in order of importance. Nonetheless, Culyer is quick to admit that the N.H.S. today does not minimize the state of ill health. Those who are most "in need" are not necessarily the ones receiving medical treatment. And Culyer, being an economist, recognizes why this is true — the behavior of British patients is governed by the demand for medical care, not by their "need" for it.

In the first place, as we have noted, a great many people are ill and do not know it. This was not only true in the 1930's, it's also true today. In the second place, even when people are aware that they are in "need" they do not necessarily seek treatment. The 1930's study found that although 26 percent of those surveyed believed they were ill, only 8 percent were actually seeking treatment.[19] More recent studies suggest that the disparity between recognized illness and the attempt to secure treatment may be even greater.[20]

In the language of economics, an individual's "demand" for a good or service is the quantity of the good or service he is willing and able to pay for. *Demand* is different from *need,* precisely because people do not necessarily demand what they need. But demand is also different from *want.* People might want something, but be unwilling to pay the price necessary to get it.

At first glance, it might seem that under British health care, "demand" and "want" become indistinguishable. After all, since health care is free to the user, the price is zero. That means that the potential patient does not have to be willing to pay anything for medical services; he only has to want it. Right? Well, that's the way Bevan envisioned it. But that's not the way it has worked.

Recall our experience with gasoline rationing in the United States. At that time the money price was low, but waiting lines were long. So in order to get gasoline, a customer had to pay for gasoline with his time as well as with his cash. In a similar way, potential consumers of health care in Britain face a great many non-cash deterrents. One of the most important of these is *time.*

The upshot is that, even under a system of "free" health care, health care is not really free — even to the users. Those patients who actually receive care have to be willing to wait longer and bear more inconveniences than other patients. In an important sense, then, the distribution of health care in Britain today is determined far more by the *demand* for health care than by the *need* for health care.

Striking testimony to this point is furnished by yet another survey of the British population.[21] The study covered a period of ten years, and compared two groups — a group of people who never saw their doctors and a group comprised of people with an average number of attendances. The rather shocking conclusion of the study was: there was little obvious medical difference in the health status of the two groups!

Health Care and Life Expectancy

One of the reasons why the technological view of health care is so appealing is that a great many people tend to view health care in terms of the critical alternative between life and death. An image quickly comes to mind of an unconscious accident victim being rushed to the emergency room of a hospital for life-saving treatment. In what sense can this patient be said to "demand" medical care? The most we can say in this case is that if the patient receives emergency care he may live. If he does not receive it, he may die. For this reason, it seems quite proper to say that in order to live, or have a reasonable chance of living, the patient "needs" medical care.

In a similar way, there are many other headline-grabbing instances in which medical care seems to represent the difference between life and death. A kidney patient, for example, "needs" renal dialysis. If he receives the treatment, he lives. If he does not, he dies. Similarly, a patient on a life-support system can be said to "need" the treatment he is receiving in order to live. If the "plug" is pulled, the patient will die. In both cases, the patients' "demand" for medical care seems largely irrelevant. If we ask what is the most they would be willing to pay for medical treatment, we are in effect asking what is the most they would be willing to pay for life! The answer is: they would probably be willing to trade their entire personal wealth in return for treatment.

The problem with these examples is that they are so misleading. It is true that immediate medical treatment may mean the difference between life and death for some patients. But such cases are actually quite rare in comparison to the broad range of medical services given to the population as a whole. In any one year, for example, only about

13 percent of British patients suffer from "life-threatening" illness.[22] Moreover, most of these patients do not require emergency care or even immediate hospitalization.

On the average, only 2.3 percent of all British patients receive in-patient care in hospitals.[23] What is more, almost half of these patients are suffering from some chronic illness, not a life-threatening illness.[24] Even among those patients who *do* require life-saving treatment, there is often little that medical science can offer beyond perhaps a short extension of the patient's life.[25] What is true for hospital services generally is also true for surgery. It is estimated that only 10 percent of all surgery involves emergency, life-or-death conditions.[26]

What all of this means is that the odds are really quite low that any particular individual will require life-saving medical treatment and then be able to resume his normal life. It happens, but not that often. The tendency to think of medical care as primarily determining the difference between life and death is reflected in the enormous attention given to mortality rates in modern times. Not long ago, life expectancy at birth was about 35 years, even in the most advanced of countries. Today, life expectancy at birth in most industrialized countries is hovering around 70 years.

What accounts for this enormous jump in average life span? The major reasons for the increase are well known. In all industrialized countries there has been a dramatic decrease in infant mortality rates[27] and in the devastating effects of infectious diseases. What role did medicine play in all of this? Apparently a very minor one.

Thomas McKeown, Professor of Social Medicine at Birmingham University (England), has made a detailed study of changes in the British death rate and their causes between 1850 and 1971.[28] His major finding is that more sanitary living conditions (pure drinking water, more sanitary sewage disposal, pasteurization of milk, etc.) were far more important in combatting infectious diseases than developments in modern medicine.

Take tuberculosis for example. Between 1850 and 1970, the British death rate from tuberculosis dropped by more than 99.5 percent. Yet the bulk of that decrease — about 86 percent - occurred before an effective drug became available in the late 1940's. Even when anti-TB drugs did become accessible, they were probably not the major reason for the continuing drop in the death rate. Another British writer, Robin Bates, argues that streptomycin may have accounted for only 3 percent of the remaining reduction in tuberculosis deaths.[29]

Typhoid is another example. Thanks to chlorination of water, better sanitation and improvement in personal hygiene, typhoid became rare before any effective drug had been developed to combat it. Much the same can be said about many of the other great plagues of the 19th century — cholera, dysentery, malaria, scarlet fever and diphtheria. In fact, Robin Bates argues that, as in the case of tuberculosis, medicine usually concentrates on the "3 percent solution."[30]

Even in those areas where the development of vaccines appears to have been a major factor in eliminating infectious disease — such as polio and smallpox — the results are more properly attributed to *medical research* rather than *medical treatment.* Smallpox, for example, is an age-old disease that once killed, blinded, or disfigured hundreds of thousands a year. Today the disease has virtually disappeared from our planet. Yet at the time of this writing there is apparently still no "cure" for smallpox.

Of all the causes of the increase in life expectancy, no single cause is as important as the decrease in infant mortality. Even today, the combined risk of death in all the years between the age of one and 20 is less than the risk of death in the first year of life.[31] For this reason, an enormous amount of research has been conducted on the causes of infant mortality and on the conditions responsible for its decline.

The results of this research have caused a rather radical revision in many experts' thinking about medical care. Not too many years ago, it was widely believed that infant mortality rates were a reliable indicator of the quality of health care received by the general population. Critics of American health care were fond of citing international comparisons of infant mortality rates. Since the United States often fared badly in these comparisons, the statistics added fuel to the charge that "capitalist" medical care is inferior to "socialist" medical care.

Today, the attitude of most researchers is quite different. In fact, many question whether medical care has *any effect at all* upon infant mortality. The reason is that, as in the case of infectious diseases, most of the improvement apparently has occurred for non-medical reasons.

Back in the 16th and 17th centuries, the infant mortality rate among Europe's ruling families was about 200 infant deaths per 1,000 live births.[32] (The rate for the population as a whole may have been two or three times as high.) By the 19th century, this rate had fallen to about 70. For those who believe that medical care had something to do with the decline, recall what the practice of medicine consisted of during that time period. Those were the days when John Donne was treated for fever by doctors who placed a dead pigeon at his feet to draw "vapours" from his brain.

Even in the 20th century, most of the improvement in infant mortality statistics appears to have been little affected by medical care. In 1900, the infant mortality rate in the United States was still quite high. (In New York City, for example, it was 140 per 1,000 live births). Yet over the next 30 years it fell at an average annual rate of 2.5 percent. Similar declines were experienced in almost every country undergoing rapid economic expansion.[33]

The reasons? Most of the decline seems to have been due to a reduction of the "diarrhea-pneumonia complex", and most experts attribute this reduction to an improvement in general living conditions. Other factors may have been important too — the income and educational level of the parents, the attitude of the mother, etc. But most researchers today attribute very little of the overall decline in infant mortality to improved medical care.

Most of the dramatic increase in life expectancy, then, has been primarily due to an improvement in the way people are living. A more sanitary environment and better personal hygiene are by far the most important factors contributing to the decline of infectious diseases and infant mortality. In some cases, the results of medical research have also been important — especially the development of vaccines. But the role of medical treatment in extending life expectancy has apparently been minor.

What is more, evidence suggests that even today the availability of medical treatment has only a marginal impact on mortality rates. In Table 4-1, we have presented some recent international statistics on infant mortality rates and per capita spending on medical care. As the table indicates, infant mortality in the U.S. is much higher than the rate in Scandinavian countries. The U.S. rate is not the highest, however; higher rates were recorded in Germany, Italy and Ireland — countries with full-blown national insurance schemes.

Few health experts today would claim that such statistics indicate a difference in the quality of medical care in these countries, however. The differences between the U.S. and the Scandinavian countries, for example, are of long standing. As Victor Fuchs has pointed out, the U.S. rate was also much higher than the rates for the

Scandinavian countries "long before medical care could have made much difference."[34]

Table 4-1

PER CAPITA SPENDING ON MEDICAL CARE, LIFE EXPECTANCY AND INFANT MORTALITY RATES, 1975

COUNTRY	PER CAPITA EXPENDITURE ON MEDICAL CARE (in 1976 U.S. dollars)	LIFE EXPECTANCY AT BIRTH	INFANT MORTALITY RATE[1] (1975)
Australia	$427	72	16.1[2]
Canada	548	73	15.5[2]
Finland	383	69	10.2[2]
France	531	73	13.6
Germany	645	71	19.7
Ireland	161	72	18.4
Italy	190	72	20.7
Japan	243	73	10.0
Netherlands	566	74	10.3
Norway	500	74	11.1
Spain	152	72	12.1
Switzerland	492	73	10.7
United Kingdom	188	72	16.0[2]
United States	593	71	16.7[2]
White			14.8[2]
Non-white			24.9[2]

1. Number of deaths under one year of age per 1,000 live births.
2. Data are for 1974.

Source: Per capita spending data reproduced from Table 3-2. Data on life expectancy taken from Population Reference Bureau, *World Population Growth and Response: 1965-1975* (Washington, D.C.: Population Reference Bureau, April, 1976), pp. 267 ff. Data on infant mortality taken from Organization for Economic Cooperation and Development, *Public Expenditure on Health* (Paris: OECD, 1977), Table 17, p. 49.

The most revealing feature of Table 4-1 is that there is virtually no relationship between per capita spending on health care and infant mortality rates. Not only is this true among countries with widely different health systems, it is also true within each of the countries themselves. In the U.S., for example, the number of infant deaths in 1970 was almost 20 per 1,000 live births. Yet the U.S. rate for whites was 17.4 and for whites in North Dakota (the most favorable state), the rate was 14.[35] Similarly, there are large differences in infant mortality rates among socioeconomic classes in Britain, despite the fact that all participate in the same N.H.S.[36]

As Table 4-2 shows, there are also wide variations among the various health regions of England. The infant mortality rates in Manchester and Liverpool, for example, are almost 40 percent higher than the rate for the South Western region.

Table 4-2

INFANT AND PERINATAL MORTALITY RATES:
UNITED KINGDOM, 1977

REGION	INFANT MORTALITY RATE[1]	PERINATAL MORTALITY RATE[2]
ENGLAND	13.7	16.9
Northern	14.9	19.1
Yorkshire	15.5	18.1
Trent	13.9	16.7
East Anglia	11.2	13.0
N.W. Thames	11.8	14.8
N.E. Thames	14.0	16.1
S.E. Thames	13.1	16.8
S.W. Thames	11.6	14.6
Wessex	13.1	15.5
Oxford	12.7	15.0
South Western	12.5	16.2
West Midlands	15.0	19.4
Mersey	14.4	18.8
North Western	14.8	18.5
WALES	13.5	17.9
SCOTLAND	16.1	18.3
N. IRELAND	17.2	21.1

1. Number of deaths under one year of age per 1,000 live births.
2. Number of deaths occurring after the 28th week of pregnancy or during the first week of life per 1,000 total births.

Source: *Royal Commission on the National Health Service Report* (Merrison Report) (London: Her Majesty's Stationery Office, 1979), Table 3.3, p. 17.

One beneficial outgrowth of all of the recent research on mortality rates is that health economists now have a much better understanding of what factors do influence mortality rates. Even today, the most important of these relate to our personal life styles. The results of one recent study are depicted in Table 4-3. Although the study was done with U.S. data, there seems to be general agreement that the results would be similar for Britain as well as other industrialized countries.[37]

Table 4-3

PERCENTAGE CHANGES IN U.S. AGE-SPECIFIC MORTALITY
RATES RESULTING FROM A 10 PERCENT INCREASE IN
SEVERAL VARIABLES

	10% Increase In:			
% Change in Mortality	Income	Education	Cigarette Consumption	Per Capita Health Expenditure
	+2.0	-2.2	+1.0	-0.65

Source: Richard Auster, Irving Leveson, and Deborah Sarachek, "The Production of
Health; an Exploratory Study," in Victor Fuchs, ed., *Essays in the
Economics of Health and Medical Care* (New York: National Bureau of
Economic Research — Columbia University Press, 1972), Table 8.3, p. 145.

One of the most interesting results of the study is that there is
a strong and positive relationship between personal income and mortality. The apparent reason for this is that many forms of consumption that are harmful to health increase as income increases. As people become wealthier, they tend to indulge in more harmful activities
— they smoke more, eat too much, consume more alcohol, drive faster cars, etc.

Increased education has an opposite influence. Better-educated
individuals tend to be better informed, and better-informed individuals tend to know more about forms of consumption that are
hazardous to their health.

The most striking result shown in Table 4-3, however, is the fact
that per capita health expenditures contribute very little to a decrease
in the mortality rate. A ten percent increase (or decrease) in spending
on health care apparently has an impact on the overall mortality rate
of less than one percent.[38]

We can now summarize two general principles concerning the
relationship between health care and life expectancy: First, most of
the health dollars spent in most industrialized countries are not spent
in ways that directly increase life expectancy. Second, insofar as
health dollars are directed toward life-saving medical treatment, the
effect on overall mortality rates is marginal.

These two principles help us understand why two different populations may have wide differences in the availability of medical resources, and yet still have similar mortality rates. They also help ex-

plain why different populations may have equal availability of medical resources and yet have very different mortality rates. And they help explain why it is so misleading to view medical care primarily in terms of the critical alternative between life and death.

Health Care and Economic Efficiency

In the most general sense, the word "efficiency" means *the property of producing or acting with a minimum amount of expense, waste and effort.* Just about every choice we make can be evaluated by the standards of efficiency. In general, the efficient choice is the choice that results in the largest benefit, given the cost — or the choice that results in the smallest cost, given the benefit we seek.

Most of us have some idea of what the term efficiency means when applied to our personal lives. We may even have some idea of what it means for a business firm to be efficient. But economists go beyond this. They not only apply the concept of efficiency to individuals and business firms, they also apply the concept to entire markets for goods and services.

In general, if a market is efficient, the total benefits created for consumers and producers will be as large as possible, given the total cost imposed on all the market participants. Similarly, if the market is efficient, the total costs imposed on consumers and producers will be as small as possible, given the total benefits that are realized in that market.

If a market is inefficient, waste exists. The existence of such waste means that, as a group, the participants in the market are less well-off than they could be. Waste, in other words, is an extra and unnecessary cost that consumers and producers have to bear. This extra cost is not necessarily distributed equally. It is often, for example, disproportionately heaped on consumers or upon certain groups of consumers, as opposed to producers. It is also often difficult to measure the cost of waste due to inefficiency.

Economists mainly agree that the concept of efficiency applies to the health care market in the same way that it applies to markets for other goods and services. Health economist Joseph Newhouse, for example, has recently argued that the formal conditions for an efficient health care market are identical to the formal conditions for efficiency in any other market.[39] What follows is a non-technical discussion of some of the necessary conditions for an efficient health care market.

The first requirement for an efficient market is: *medical services must be produced at a minimum cost.* This requirement is almost intuitively self-evident. If the cost of producing health care services is not minimized, waste will clearly exist. But what is not obvious to many non-specialists is that in the health care market there are often many different ways of achieving the same result.

Varicose veins, for example, may be treated with injection therapy or by surgery. Renal failure may be treated by dialysis or by a kidney transplant. A great many types of treatment may be performed equally well in a hospital, a community health center, or in a general practitioner's office. Indeed, the options open to us in the delivery of medical care are almost infinite. The standard of efficiency, however, requires that we choose the lowest-cost option out of the many options that are available.

It might seem that the goal of efficiency in production is unobjectionable. How could anyone quarrel with it? Why would anyone willingly choose to produce inefficiently? The problem is: as individuals, we inevitably tend to respond to *personal* costs and benefits, not *social* costs and benefits. One of the virtues of a free, competitive market is that personal and social costs and benefits tend to coincide. Producers, in search of personal profit, have an incentive to keep production costs as low as possible. Those producers who are the most successful at minimizing costs are also the ones who are able to most successfully compete for consumers by keeping prices low.

These incentives are often absent, however, when the market is not allowed to work. In creating the N.H.S., the British government abolished competition among the suppliers of medical care by creating a virtual monopoly. In addition, it is a non-profit monopoly owned and operated by the government. Under these conditions, personal costs and benefits very often diverge from social costs and benefits.

In recent years, economists have devoted considerable attention to the reasons for this phenomenon.[40] The conclusions of this research are loosely formulated in "Friedman's Law": Anything produced by government can be produced by private industry at one-half the cost.[41] Friedman's Law seems to describe fairly accurately the difference between private and public production in the areas of garbage collection, fire protection, education, postal service and in a great many other areas. In the following chapters, we will look at a great many examples of that law at work in the health care market.

Part of the process of production is the mechanism by which goods and services are physically distributed to consumers. A natural corollary of our first requirement for an efficient market, then, is: *medical services must be physically distributed to consumers at a minimum cost.* Most schemes of non-price rationing violate this principle with abandon.

In the gasoline market, for example, rationing by waiting in line does not produce additional gasoline. Nor does it produce additional income for the market participants taken as a group. But it does impose an unnecessary and wasteful cost on consumers — the cost of hours spent waiting.[42] In a similar way, rationing by waiting in the health care market violates the standard of efficiency. The extra costs imposed by such a system can be enormous.

A second requirement for an efficient market is: *the value of medical services rendered to each consumer must be at least equal to the cost of producing those services.* To illustrate this principle, imagine that a patient is eligible for a surgical procedure which costs $1,000 to perform. Now suppose we give the patient a choice between having the operation or receiving $1,000 in cash. If the patient chooses to have the operation, we may infer that the operation is at least worth $1,000 to him. On the other hand, if the patient opts for the cash, we may infer that the value of the operation is less than its cost — in this case, performing the operation would be inefficient, and, therefore, wasteful.

In most private markets this principle is easily satisfied. Prices generally reflect costs of production, and consumers do not buy goods and services unless they expect the value of what they receive to be at least as great as the money price they have to pay. But when money prices are absent, a real problem exists. When medical services are made free to the user at the time they are consumed, ample opportunities exist for the principle to be violated.

In the N.H.S., for example, a $1,000 operation is theoretically offered to patients at a price of zero. This means that even if the patient places a very low value on the operation, say $50, the patient will still demand it — even though $950 worth of waste will be created.

A special problem, though, arises in the health care market, and in some other markets as well. British health economist Anthony Culyer argues that consumption of medical care is not entirely an individual act.[43] That is because, according to Culyer, we care about the medical treatment received by others. So even though the patient values his own operation at only $50, other members of the community may value that operation at an additional $950 or more. Why?

Because they are not disinterested; they "care."

There are several problems with Culyer's argument. Although it is no doubt true that, both in Britain and the United States people care in the abstract about the medical treatment received by their neighbors, it is not clear *how much* they care. As we shall see in Chapter 6, the N.H.S. allows a great many patients to die because the cost of their treatment is judged to be too high. Yet there does not seem to be much public outrage; and, indeed, there seems to be little political pressure to acquire expensive and potentially life-saving technology that has recently been made available to U.S. citizens.

Another problem with this argument is that, even if people care very much about the health care received by others, surely they would prefer to give priority to those who are most in need. Yet, as we shall see, most observers believe that the N.H.S. is characterized by the "Inverse Care Law": those who receive the most medical care are those who need it the least. We argued in Chapter 2 that the N.H.S. was not founded in order to redistribute medical care to those who needed it the most. Nor is there any significant political pressure to do so today.

The upshot is that non-price rationing of medical care in Britain furnishes powerful incentives to violate the second requirement for economic efficiency. We will encounter many specific examples of such violations in the following chapters.

A third requirement for an efficient market is: *medical services provided should be distributed among consumers so as to maximize their social value.* In other words, goods and services produced should go to their highest-valued uses. In the private marketplace this requirement is almost always satisfied. The price system is fully comparable to an auction. Given that goods and services are available for consumption, market prices ensure that those who actually do consume them are those who place the highest value on them.

An example of the importance of this principle in the gasoline market may be helpful: suppose that I have a gallon of gasoline that I value at $1, while you would be willing to pay as much as $2 for it. In order to achieve efficiency, I must be allowed to sell my gasoline to you. If the sale is not allowed, economic waste results. In this example, the amount of the waste is equal to $1. The example helps to explain why most economists are so critical of rationing gasoline by the policy of first come/first served. Such a policy can be enormously wasteful because it contains no mechanism for shifting gasoline to those uses where it has the highest value.

The principle works in a similar way in the market for health care. True, in this market, as in the gasoline market, we may not always want ability to pay to be a constraint. That is, we may want to subsidize the consumption of low-income individuals. But this desire need not prevent us from allocating health care efficiently.

Each year the N.H.S. spends millions of dollars providing free contraceptives to the public. It spends millions more subsidizing the consumption of tranquilizers, sleeping pills, tonics and vitamins. At the same time, literally thousands wait for months and even years in constant pain because important medical services are in short supply. Indeed, even the most ardent defenders of socialized medicine do not claim that in Britain health services flow to their highest-valued uses.

By violating these requirements for an efficient health care market, the N.H.S. causes British citizens to bear extra, unnecessary costs. It thus makes them less well off than they could be. The consequences of violating the first requirement are that the British do not get their money's worth for their tax dollars. They have less care and a lower quality of care than could be achieved for the same amount of spending. The consequence of violating the second requirement is that what care they do receive is often less valuable than other goods and services that could have been provided with the same money. The consequence of violating the third requirement is that many of the most valuable uses of health care spending are foregone, leaving a great many people living in pain for long periods of time — and sometimes leaving them without hope of medical care at all.

The concept of economic efficiency, then, is crucially important in evaluating the British system of socialized medicine. In terms of budgetary costs, the cost of British health care is among the lowest in the industrialized world. But when non-budgetary costs are included — including the costs of inferior quality care, the costs of waiting, and the costs of pain, suffering and even death borne by those patients and their families who are denied medical care — the cost of British health care actually delivered may well be the highest in the industrialized world.

Footnotes

1. In practice, some people actually specialized in waiting. For a fee they agreed to wait in line and have your car filled with gasoline. Motorists who took advantage of such arrangements thus avoided the waiting costs. But after paying someone else to wait for them, they probably paid considerably more than 85 cents per gallon.

2. A review of a number of these studies, along with a rigorous economic analysis of the theory of the demand for medical care, is contained in Joseph P. Newhouse, *The Economics of Medical Care* (Reading, Mass.: Addison-Wesley, 1978), Ch. 2.

3. Michael H. Cooper, *Rationing Health Care* (New York: Halstead Press, 1975), p. 25.

4. Economic Models, Ltd., *The British Health Care System* (Chicago: American Medical Association, 1975), p. 106.

5. *Ibid*, p. 107.

6. Roger I. Lee and Lewis W. Jones, *The Fundamentals of Good Medical Care: An Outline of the Fundamentals of Good Medical Care and an Estimate of the Service Required to Supply the Medical Needs of the United States* (Chicago, Ill.: University of Chicago Press, 1933).

7. Hyman K. Schonfield, Jean F. Heston, and Isadore S. Falk, "Number of Physicians Required for Primary Medical Care," *New England Journal of Medicine,* 286, No. 11 (March 16, 1972), pp. 571-576.

8. J. Enoch Powell, *Medicine and Politics: 1975 and After* (New York: Pitman Publishing, 1976), p. 28.

9. *Ibid,* pp. 26-27.

10. Anthony J. Culyer, *Need and the National Health Service* (Totowa, New Jersey: Rowman and Littlefield, 1976), p. 5.

11. Cited in Culyer, *Ibid,* p. 19.

12. W.P.D. Logan and E. Brooke, *Survey of Sickness 1943-1951* (London: Her Majesty's Stationery Office, 1957).

13. M.E.J. Wadsworth, R. Blaney and W.J.H. Butterfield, *Health and Sickness: the Choice of Treatment* (Tavistock Press, 1971); and K. Dunnell and A. Cartwright, *Medicine Takers, Prescribers and Hoarders* (London: Routledge and Kegan Paul, 1972).

14. Cited in Cooper, *Rationing Health Care,* p. 13

15. Ruth Levitt, *The Reorganized National Health Service,* (London: Croom Helm, Ltd., 1976), n.6, p. 236.

16. For an interesting glimpse at the future possibilities in this field, see Jerome Tucille, *Here Comes Immortality* (New York: Stein and Day, 1973).

17. For a survey of recent advances in scanner technology, see Boyce Rensberger, "New Views into Body Aid Diagnosis," *New York Times,* November 14, 1978.

18. Culyer, *Need and the National Health Service,* p. 7.

19. *Ibid,* p. 5

20. Cooper, *Rationing Health Care,* pp. 11-13

21. N. Kessel and M. Sheppard, "The Health Attitudes of People Who Seldom Consult a Doctor," *Medical Care,* 3, no. 6, 1965.

22. Levitt, *The Reorganized National Health Service,* p. 95.

23. *Ibid,* p. 179.

24. *Ibid,* p. 199.

25. In 1964-65, over 20 percent of U.S. hospital expenditures on individuals over 25 years of age were made on behalf of individuals in the last year of life. Newhouse estimates that the figure today is probably from 25 to 35 percent, and perhaps even more. See Newhouse, *The Economics of Medical Care,* p. 84.

26. J. Bunker, "Risks and Benefits of Surgery," in Office of Health Economics, *Benefits and Risks in Medical Care, 1974.*

27. Infant mortality rates record the number of deaths in the first year of life per 1,000 live births.

28. Thomas McKeown, "A Historic Appraisal of the Medical Task," in McKeown, et. al., *Medical History and Medical Care* (London: Oxford University Press for the Nuffield Provincial Hospitals Trust, 1971). See also, T. McKeown and R.G. Record, "Reasons for the Decline of Mortality in England and Wales during the Nineteenth Century," *Population Studies,* vol. 16, 1962.
29. Cited in George Will, "A Right to Health?", *Newsweek*, August 7, 1978, p. 88.
30. *Ibid.*
31. Victor Fuchs, *Who Shall Live?* (New York: Basic Books, 1974), p. 40.
32. Sigismund Teller, "Birth and Death among Europe's Ruling Families since 1500," in D.J. Glass and D.E.C. Eversley, eds., *Population in History,* (London: Edward Arnold, 1965), pp. 87-100.
33. Fuchs, *Who Shall Live?,* p. 32.
34. *Ibid*, p. 38.
35. *Ibid*, pp. 37-38.
36. *Ibid*, p. 34.
37. See Culyer, *Need and the National Health Service.*
38. Warning: it would be incorrect to infer from these results the probable effects of eliminating all the doctors, nurses and hospitals from a country. If we eliminated all medical treatment, the increase in mortality might be quite substantial. What Table 4-3 *does* show is the probable effect of altering per capita health care expenditures within the range likely to be considered.
39. Newhouse, *The Economics of Medical Care*, Ch.6.
40. See, for example, John Goodman and Edwin Dolan, *The Economics of Public Policy: The Micro View* (St. Paul: West Publishing Co., 1979), Ch.6.
41. David Friedman, *The Machinery of Freedom* (New Rochelle, New York: Arlington House, 1978).
42. For an analysis of the cost of waiting in the gasoline market, see Goodman and Dolan, *Economics of Public Policy*, Ch.3.
43. Culyer, *Need and the National Health Service*, p. 89.

Chapter 5
Rationing: The General Practitioner

The Role of the Family Doctor

A good place to begin our inquiry into medical rationing is with the general practitioner. Britain's 26,000 general practitioners have been described as the "front line of the N.H.S."[1] For most patients, the general practitioner represents the gateway into the vast range of services offered by the N.H.S. — the pharmaceutical services, the hospital services, and local authority services such as health visitors and home nurses. What is more, 90 percent of all episodes of sickness handled by the N.H.S. are dealt with from start to finish by the general practitioner.[2]

Over 97 percent of Britain's population are registered with a G.P. under the N.H.S.[3] Patients are generally free to choose their physician, and in large cities a considerable range of choice may exist. But doctors are also free to refuse patients; and just as patients may switch doctors, doctors retain the right to have patients removed from their lists.

On the average, the patient list for a general practitioner numbers about 2,351. Some doctors serve a much larger number, however. It is estimated that 14 percent of general practitioners are responsible for 3,000 or more patients.[4] Once a patient is on a doctor's list, the doctor is responsible for all "primary medical care." But, as we shall see, what constitutes "primary care" differs considerably from physician to physician.

One of the most interesting aspects of general practitioner care is the fact that in Britain doctors make house calls. A general practitioner, in principle, is responsible for 24-hour-a-day service to the patients on his list. Thus, in principle, a doctor's work-week is 168 hours long — a fact which is often mentioned when complaints are registered by general practitioners over the level of remuneration they receive.

The central problem that arises in general practitioner care is the same problem that pervades the entire N.H.S. The demand for care is virtually infinite, while the supply of care is quite limited. The problem at the general practitioner level has been exacerbated by two factors. First, although the ratio of patients to *all* doctors has fallen since 1949, the ratio of patients to general practitioners has actually increased.[5] (See Figure 5-1.) Second, the quantity of services delivered by general practitioners appears to have declined even more. Over the last decade, home visits by general practitioners have been reduced by 60 percent, and the number of office visits by patients has been reduced by 15 percent.[6]

Figure 5-1

RATIO OF PATIENTS TO DOCTORS

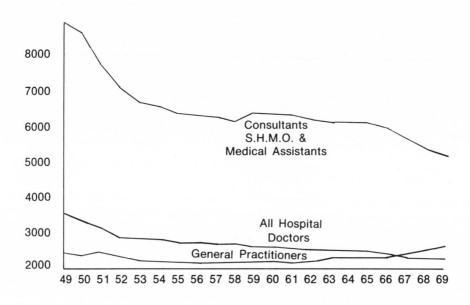

9000
Registered
Patients per
Doctor (w.t.e.)

Note: w.t.e. = whole time equivalent
Source: Economic Models, Ltd. *The British Health Care System* (Chicago: American Medical Association, 1976), Figure 5.1, p. 79.

How, then, do the British ration the services of general practitioners? Let us look first at the behavior of the patients.

Who Demands Care?

As we saw in Chapter 4, one of the most important economic principles governing the market for health care is the law of demand. The demand for health care varies with the price charged to the user, and the lower the price, the greater the quantity that will be demanded.

When medical services are potentially available with no charge to the user of those services, patients potentially face a price equal to zero. Under these conditions, each patient has an incentive to consume medical services so long as those services have a personal value slightly greater than zero. This means that each and every service general practitioners can provide will be demanded by patients so long as those services have some positive value.

To the typical patient, then, the incentives are quite clear. Since the doctor's services are free, why not consult him for every illness, for every problem — no matter how insignificant? Why not visit the doctor even if there is no apparent illness, just to make sure everything checks out all right? Evidence suggests that this is precisely what patients do. The vast proportion of the G.P.'s work is concerned with the routine, the non-urgent, and often the non-medical.

One study found that in 1966, one-half of the doctors surveyed felt that more than 25 percent of their consultations were for "trivial, unnecessary, or inappropriate reasons."[7] Of these "trivial" consultations, 53 percent were for such conditions as coughs, colds, morning sickness, dandruff, indigestion and the like. Another 18 percent of these visits were made only to obtain the doctor's signature on a certificate of illness or other official form — and no medical treatment was sought.

General practitioners are called upon to act as social workers for the lonely, to give advice on the rearing of wayward offspring, and to sign the backs of passport photos. A 1974 study found that 28 percent of consultations were for such non-medical services.[8] Of the remaining 72 percent who actually sought treatment, in 43 percent of the cases the doctor was unable to diagnose any definite illness. Most of these "recovered," however, after some reassurance and an occasional placebo. Various other studies have estimated that from 30 to 75 percent of consultations "are with patients displaying no objective evidence (either psychological or physical) for their attendance."[9]

One of the difficulties of relying too heavily on the results of these studies is that they record medical *opinion*, rather than medical *fact*. The very serious ailment is likely to present itself to the general practitioner very rarely. He is likely to see only one case of cervical cancer in three years; only one brain tumor in ten years.[10] As a result, the average general practitioner may be notoriously unskilled at diagnosing certain types of serious illness. On top of that, as we shall see, the conditions under which most patients are examined increase the likelihood that a more subtle form of illness, no matter how serious, will go undetected in the G.P.'s office.

Nonetheless, there is considerable independent evidence to corroborate the trivial nature of a great many G.P. consultations. Take sickness certificates, for example. These are necessary in order to legitimize absences from work and often qualify the patient for government sickness benefits. As Table 5-1 indicates, there is considerable evidence that dissatisfaction with work may be a principal determinant of "sickness." As the table shows, almost twice as many sick days were taken by those dissatisfied with their work as by those who were satisfied.

Table 5-1

DAYS OFF WORK PER PERSON PER YEAR
AND WORK SATISFACTION

	Males	**Females**	**Total**
Very or Fairly Satisfied	7.8	6.4	7.3
Neither	9.3	6.2	8.3
Rather or Very Dissatisfied	13.1	18.3	13.1
Total	8.1	6.9	7.7

Source: General Household Survey, *Introductory Report*, (London: Her Majesty's Stationery Office, 1973).

Cooper argues that sickness certificates tend to be a "medical euphemism rather than a clinical opinion," and that "periods of absence probably reflect the generosity of current sickness benefits as much as thresholds of sickness."[11] In 1960, a worker earning an average wage could collect 40 percent of his normal pay when off work for two weeks or more for reasons of illness. By 1969, a worker earning a comparable wage could collect 70 percent of his normal salary for the same reason. Workers have apparently responded to these incentives in a predictable way. Between 1958 and 1969, days of incapacity per person increased 26 percent for men and 11 percent for women. New spells of incapacity per one hundred people increased 44 percent for men and 45 percent for women.[12] In 1975, about 2.3 percent of Britain's labor force was absent from work for reason of ill health at any one time. By contrast, absenteeism due to sickness was only 1.6 percent in U.S. labor markets that year.[13]

Other evidence of the increasing triviality of G.P. consultations comes from the Royal College of General Practitioners surveys of morbidity.[14] Between 1955-56 and 1970-71, there was a general increase in episodes of illness presented to general practitioners.[15] But over the same time period there was a decrease in the number of consultations per episode. Furthermore, the number of people who failed to consult a doctor and the number of episodes of serious ailments remained constant.

The fact that a great many claims on the G.P. are for services that are trivial, non-urgent and even non-medical does not mean that the more serious claims have already been catered to. In the competition for the doctor's services, the trivial competes with the urgent. The medical competes with the non-medical. To see how this competition affects the quality of care patients actually receive, we need to look more closely at the position of the doctor.

The Supply of General Practitioner Services

Former Minister of Health Enoch Powell once wrote that "one of the most striking features of the N.H.S. is the continual deafening chorus of complaining which arises day after night from every part of it.[16] One area where the complaints have been especially deafening is the area of general practitioner service.

From the earliest days of the N.H.S. general practitioners faced an almost impossible task — to provide high quality care for those who sought it. With G.P. services free to the user, the demand for these services soared. Doctors watched helplessly as their waiting rooms became packed with potential patients, each willing to wait until his turn arrived. The choices were two-fold: First, the doctor could retain his professional standards and continue to provide the quality of care he had always provided. This, of course, would mean that a majority of those in the waiting room would either be sent home or would leave voluntarily out of frustration as the doctor worked long into the night. Second, the doctor could do what many service station attendants did during the U.S. gasoline shortage a few years back — try to provide partial service to as many patients as possible.

Many doctors chose the second option, and the results have been dramatic. Whereas G.P.s in the U.S. spend about 13 minutes with each patient,[17] on the average, in Britain the time spent with each patient is less than five minutes.[18] To appreciate what this means, consider the fact that a doctor occasionally must surely see a patient with a serious ailment. For the truly serious case, the doctor may well spend 15 to 30 minutes on the examination. But this in turn means that he must be spending as little as one or two minutes with most of his other patients in order to keep the average down to five minutes.

Apparently very few doctors exceed the five minute average by much. A recent survey revealed that only 11 percent of the G.P.s devoted more than six minutes to each patient, on the average.[19] Moreover, balanced against those who devote above-average time to their patients, there are those who are well below the average. One doctor recently admitted that, while practicing in Britain, he was "reduced to seeing twenty-four patients per hour."[20] That's two and one-half minutes per patient!

Not having enough time to adequately examine patients is one of the most common and bitter complaints of British general practitioners. A 1968 survey disclosed that 68 percent of all G.P.s regard this as a very serious or fairly serious problem in general practice.[21] "Not enough time *ever* to do one's work adequately and still have time to live a normal family life,"[22] is a representative comment. Still others complain that their office has been reduced "to the status of a production line."[23]

Of course, the more conscientious a doctor, the more frustrating these experiences will be. A great many doctors, however, have become considerably less conscientious. Dr. Derrick Henderson explains why: "I've seen colleagues change from those who opposed the government and its destruction of their doctor-patient relationship, through a transition period where despite the system they tried to do their best for their patient, to a final situation where they accepted, enjoyed, and even exploited the conditions."[24]

Dr. Henderson, as it turns out, had an opportunity to witness unconscientious medicine first hand, as a patient. Henderson, a recent immigrant from Britain, needed a medical examination by another doctor to qualify him for entry into the U.S. As an experiment, however, Henderson neglected to tell the examiner that he himself was a doctor.

The chest examination covered an area exposed by undoing the top button of his shirt. As Henderson recounts the incident,[25]

The stethoscope slid sideways like a crab marginally towards my left clavicle. I surmised the chest examination was over and now my heart was commanding my doctor's attention. Ten seconds later my abdomen was prodded as I sat dressed in the chair, and I was dismissed, the examination over.

The buzzer sounded to make the next patient come forth, and as he passed me, I noted he already had his tie off and his top button unfastened. He either was a quick learner or was already used to the system.

In Britain, you have a rushed physician and an unsophisticated patient to whom any form of laying-on of the hands or instrument is awe inspiring. You have cold weather, cold waiting rooms, and buttoned-up clothing.

It might seem that for the conscientious doctor there is another way. Why not cut down the list size? With fewer patients, a higher quality of care could be given to each one of them. While some G.P.s might be able to do this, all clearly cannot do so. That would leave most of the population without the services of a general practitioner — something the N.H.S. would never stand for. So in practice, if one doctor reduces his lists size, the list of some other doctors will simply grow by an equal amount.

But there is a more fundamental reason why most doctors do not try to reduce the number of patients on their list. The reason is financial.

The Financial Incentives of General Practitioners

By U.S. standards, the salaries of British doctors are quite low. Precisely what a G.P. can expect to earn is unclear. As of April, 1974, official estimates place the average G.P. salary at about $11,600.[26] A recent study, however, estimated that a "progressive" general practitioner could expect to earn a little under $16,000.[27] This is a doctor who handles an above average list size, works in an "under-doctored" area, and undertakes part-time hospital work. Whatever the actual figure, it is a source of bitter complaint among Britain's general practitioners. Sixty-four percent regard the level of their compensation to be a very serious, or fairly serious, problem in general practice.[28]

More important than the level of salary, however, are the financial incentives faced by the average G.P. General practitioners have every financial incentive to provide mediocre, even inferior, medical care to their patients. The doctor who would strive for excellence can do so only at considerable personal loss.

Table 5-2
HOW GENERAL PRACTITIONERS ARE PAID

Approximate % of Gross Payments to General Practitioners for General Medical Services		Schedule of fees laid down at 1st April, 1974.
19%	Basic Practice Allowance	£2,100 per annum for practices with lists in excess of 1,000 patients per doctor proportionately reduced for lists with less than 1,000 per doctor.
39%	Standard Capitation Fees	
	a. For each patient aged under 65	£1.60 per annum
	b. For each patient aged over 65	£2.30 per annum
	Payments for out of hours responsibilities (for undertaking responsibility for a list of patients at night and weekends).	
4.0%	a. Supplementary practice allowance	£400 per annum on the same basis as the Basic Practice Allowance.
4.0%	b. Supplementary and capitation fees for each patient in excess of 1,000 on the list.	£0.20 per annum
—	c. Fee for a vist requested and made between midnight and 7.00 a.m.	£3.00 per visit
	Additions to the basic practice allowance	
2.0%	a. For practice in "designated" areas (areas defined as under doctored).	£519 - £849 per annum
2.0%	b. For practicing in a group of three or more doctors	£270 per annum
4.0%	c. For seniority	Grades: i. £260 per annum ii. £520 per annum iii. £640 per annum
—	d. For the employment of an assistant.	£660 or £930 per annum
—	e. For vocational training (for five years after completion of an approved post graduate training course).	£175 per annum
6.0%	Provision of full maternity medical services by a practitioner on the obstetric list.	£22.30 per case
1.0%	Rural practice payments paid to doctors having widespread practices	Individually assessed
5.0%	Direct reimbursement for ancillary staff.	70% of remuneration of up to two whole time staff per doctor.
4.0%	Direct reimbursements of expenses incurred in providing practice accommodation.	Either actual rents paid or notional rents of premises owned by the doctor.
3.0%	Miscellaneous other payments such as post graduate training allowances, fees for vaccination and immunization, cervical cytology tests, temporary residents, emergency treatment, administration of anesthetics, arrest of dental hemorrhages, trainee practitioners, initial practice allowances, inducement payments, payments during sickness, practice premises improvement grants, group practice loans, etc.	

Source: Economic Models, Ltd., *The British Health Care System* (Chicago: American Medical Association, 1976), pp. 83-84, Table 5-3. Reprinted with the permission of the American Medical Association.

Table 5-2 gives some indication of why this is true. General practitioners receive a basic practice allowance and a standard capitation fee — a set amount per patient. The fee is higher for patients over 65 years of age (on the theory that the medical needs of these patients are above average). There is also some adjustment for practicing in "under-doctored" areas, and additional compensation for certain types of services rendered.

The most crucial thing to note, however, is that doctors are primarily paid according to the number of patients on their list. They are not paid for the quality or quantity of services rendered. This means that a doctor has a financial incentive to expand his list size.[29]But he has little incentive to improve the quality of service he renders. As Enoch Powell describes it, "Whether the practitioner is good . . . or indifferent, he gets the same remuneration for the same list."[30]

What all of this means to the general practitioner is this: he gets paid for simply having a patient on his list. He gets paid the same amount whether the patient never sets foot in his door or whether the patient is a chronic who pops in every week. He gets paid the same amount whether he provides high quality care or the cursory type of examination that was given to Dr. Henderson.

There are, of course, certain minimal standards. Failure to attend to a patient, for example, is regarded as unprofessional conduct. If such a complaint is substantiated, the G.P. may be disciplined by the Medical Practices Committee which administers the G.P. service. In general, however, the N.H.S. has granted the G.P. his "clinical freedom": the right to practice medicine in accordance with his professional conscience. And instances where G.P.s are actually disciplined appear to be rare.

What is more, most British doctors appear to have little to fear from malpractice suits. In 1973 the average British physician could obtain insurance to cover legal costs and damages for about $60 a year. By contrast, insurance rates in the U.S. about that time were as high as $20,000 in some fields of surgery. Some U.S. anaesthetists were paying as much as $34,000.[31]

How have general practitioners responded to the incentive structure created by the N.H.S.? There appears to be wide variation in the responses of doctors. Studies have shown, for example, that some see twice as many patients as others with the same list size.[32]Wide variations also exist in the number of prescriptions written, the number of housecalls made, numbers of referals to specialists, and in just about every other aspect of their work that can be quantified and compared.[33]

There are, however, some general characteristics of G.P. practice that are clearly the results of the incentives that all doctors face. We have already seen that, out of necessity, G.P.s have substantially reduced the time spent with each patient. We can now add an extra bit of insight. It is clearly in the doctor's interest to reduce the time spent with each patient. After all, he receives the same salary whether he spends ten minutes, five minutes or even one minute with each patient. Time spent per patient, then, may be only partly due to the demands placed on doctors by their patients. It may also be due to the fact that the doctor has no incentive to spend much time with them.

It is precisely for this reason that we can appreciate another fact about general practice — doctors have no incentive to treat patients with serious or chronic medical problems. They have every reason to prefer the trivial to the non-trivial, the non-urgent to the urgent, the non-medical to the medical. For it is precisely the unimportant demand that can be dealt with swiftly, placing only limited burdens upon the doctor's time and medical expertise.

This is not to say that doctors prefer a waiting room full of trivial problems. They have an incentive to reduce this part of their caseload too. Some doctors believe they can educate their patients and discourage visits for inconsequential reasons.[34] Others have resorted to an appointments system — an increasingly popular technique among British G.P.s.

Under the appointments system, patients do not simply come to the doctor's office and wait their turn. Instead, they must have an appointment in advance of their visit. For most British patients the appointments system means about a three day wait before they can see their doctor, and about a two hour wait in the doctor's office if they show up for their appointment on time.[35] One advantage of the system is that it cuts down on waiting time in the doctor's office.[36] A disadvantage is that the patient who wakes up in pain is often not interested in waiting for three days before he can secure treatment.

Today, about 60 percent of G.P.s use an appointments system (as opposed to only 6 percent in 1961).[37] Moreover, there is evidence that the system actually does cut down the number of patient consultations. It probably does so for two reasons: First, many patients no doubt "recover" on their own over the three day waiting period. Second, if the patient really wants immediate attention, he can circumvent the G.P. altogether and go directly to a hospital emergency room. This is an option we will consider more fully later.

On those occasions when the doctor does see a serious or potentially serious case, he has an incentive to take advantage of another option: referral of the patient to a specialist. In general, the G.P. has no hospital privileges, and once a patient is referred to a specialist, the G.P.'s role in the treatment is essentially over. So if the patient appears to be truly ill, or if he insists that he is truly ill, why waste time on an extensive examination? Why not quickly dispose of the case by a referral?

Do general practitioners actually abuse the system in this way? There is evidence that many do. But there also appears to be wide variations in procedures used by different doctors. One study of 94 doctors found that three referred less than five patients per one thousand consultations while, at the other extreme, one doctor referred 115 per 1,000.[38] Another study of general practice in Edinburgh found the variation in referral rates ranged from .6 to 25.8 percent.[39]

A follow-up study actually examined the nature of these referrals and could find no explanation for these wide variations.[40] What is more, the study also found that 83 percent of the patients referred to specialists received no treatment other than an initial interview — that is, no pathological or X-ray investigation was made.

British health economist Michael Cooper speculates that there is another way in which doctors cut down on their work load — they substitute drugs for a rigorous examination of their patient's complaints. As Cooper explains it, "doctors may be tempted to use Librium and Valium, for example, as effective ways of cutting a consulation short."[41] The harm done may be considerable. Various studies suggest that five out of every 100 patients admitted to British hospitals are ill from some condition that was caused, at least in part, by a drug.[42] This may help explain why other surveys find that as many as one-third of all patients fail to take the drugs that are prescribed.[43]

Finally, there is a rather decisive way in which a general practitioner might cut down on his work load — he might simply fail to go to his office at all. An extreme example of this type of behavior was uncovered by the (London) *Times* a few years ago. Reporters for the *Times* attempted to contact a doctor who maintained three offices in Ellswick. As the *Times* reported the incident,

> We tried to contact a doctor there at 11:30 one Thursday morning. Out telephone call was referred, by the operator, to an emergency night number. We rang the second of the three [offices] which the doctor uses. Again, an operator intercepted the call, but this time referred us to the ... number we had previously rung. A call to the doctor's third [office] was not answered or intercepted at all. At 11:45 we rang the emer-

gency service. They said they were unable to contact the doctor, and we should have to ring him during [office] hours. When we asked when that was, the emergency service said they didn't know.[44]

The incident should be regarded as an extreme case, not a typical one. Nonetheless, it does not appear that the *Times* reporters had to search long to find such a case. And if the reporters were unable to locate the doctor, is it likely that his patients were more succesful?

As we saw in Chapter 4, it is difficult to make a quantitative assessment of how the quality of medical care has been altered by the incentive structure erected by the N.H.S. Morbidity and mortality tables are unreliable indicators of the quality of care received precisely because social and economic factors appear to be the dominant influences on both sickness and death.

Table 5-3, though, gives some idea of the quality (and the variation in quality) of services rendered by general practitioners. Doctors were asked what procedures they used when the opportunity arose. As the table indicates, a fifth of the G.P.s do not strap sprains most of the time. Two-fifths do not ordinarily stitch cuts or do vaginal examinations with a speculum. One-half do not ordinarily open abcesses. Amazingly, 65 percent never use a laryngoscope.

Another indicator is the testimony of the doctors themselves. Dr. Derrick Henderson recalls the case of a pediatrician who stopped using thermometers after the N.H.S. started. The explanation? As Henderson recalls the conversation, his colleague explained: "Takes too much time, old chap. But I do use them on occasion if a mother chatters too much and slows me down. I pop my thermometer in her mouth." Henderson also recalls how another colleague diagnosed possible appendicitis by phone: "Put your hand in your pocket, press, and if it hurts, go to the emergency room. Oh, but be sure it's your right hand," he told the patient.[45]

Financial Incentives and Other Aspects of General Practice

Former Minister of Health Enoch Powell has described the dilemma facing the British general practitioner in the following way:

The situation of the family doctor, therefore, combines private enterprise and state service without the characteristic advantages of either. The doctor cannot build up a practice and a reputation that enables him to reap the reward of his efforts either in income or in satisfaction. Paradoxically, the

Table 5-3

ACTIONS TAKEN BY DOCTORS ON CERTAIN PROCEDURES

Undertakes procedure in their practice:	Strap sprains	Excise simple cysts	Open abscesses	Stitch cuts	Do vaginal examination with speculum	Estimate haemoglobin with a haemoglobino-meter	Use of laryngoscope
	%	%	%	%	%	%	%
More often than not	80	29	52	60	60	12	9
Occasionally	18	33	42	34	28	15	26
Never	2	38	6	6	12	73	65

Source: Ann Cartwright, Patients and Their Doctors (New York: Atherton Press, 1967), p. 19, Table 4.

better he does his work, the worse off he is. The money he spends on improving his premises, providing himself with modern equipment, paying for efficient reception, clerical and other administrative staff, will not increase his earnings by one penny. On the contrary, the cost will come out of an income that would have been undiminished if he spent on none of these things. If he restricts his list to the number of patients he can treat properly and conscientiously, and devotes to consultation the amount of time and care he considers to be required . . . he will merely end up with a lower income than his less able or scrupulous fellows . . . The essence of the private enterprise system, competition for gain, has been gouged out of family doctoring, while leaving an empty shell."[46]

Powell's description is not quite correct today, at least in one respect. As Table 5-2 shows, G.P.s do get reimbursements for part of the salaries of their nurses and other assistants. Moreover, efficient use of ancilliary staff has been enhanced by the tendency toward group practice. Over 45 percent of Britain's G.P.s are now practicing in groups of three or more.[47] Even so, in 1969 only 41 percent of doctors surveyed had direct access to the services of a nurse.[48] Among doctors practicing outside of a group, 74 percent did not have access to a nurse.

A more serious problem concerns the lack of equipment to which the G.P. has access. Dr. Robert Lefever, who practices in South Kensington, provides an example of how stingy the N.H.S. can be. Dr. LeFever, it seems, wanted to install X-ray equipment in his office. He was even willing to pay for the cost of the equipment and its maintenance provided the N.H.S. would pay for the film (each film costs about $2). The government said no — confirming Dr. Lefever's feeling that "the emphasis in the health service hierarchy is always on cost rather than on quality."[49]

One reason why office equipment is so important is that a great many G.P.s in Britain simply do not have access to many diagnostic procedures. As Table 5-4 shows, only 72 percent have access to full-sized chest X-rays. Only 61 percent have access to bone and joint X-rays. Twenty-four percent have access to glucose tolerance tests, and only 19 percent have access to an electro-cardiogram.

Not only does a doctor have no financial incentive to furnish his office with diagnostic equipment, he also has no financial incentive to use such equipment when it is available, say, through a local hospital.

Table 5-4

REPORTED ACCESS TO AND USE OF VARIOUS DIAGNOSTIC PROCEDURES AMONG A SAMPLE OF DOCTORS IN ENGLAND AND WALES

Procedures	Reported Access	Reported Use of Procedures in Previous Two Weeks
	%	%
Hemoglobin	87	80
Red blood cell count	77	70
White blood cell count	75	67
Full-size chest X-rays	72	67
Bacteriologic examination of urine	65	57
Routine urinalysis	62	53
Bone and joint X-rays	61	57
Erythrocye sedimentation rate	57	48
Blood sugar	29	21
Prothrombin activity	27	20
Glucose tolerance tests	24	15
Liver function tests	24	16
Serum cholesterol	23	15
Electrocardiogram	19	15
Serum electrolytes	18	10
Blood culture	12	4
CSF micro and culture and chemistry	7	1
Radioactive iodine	6	3
B.M.R.	5	2

Source: D. Mechanic, "General Practice in England and Wales," *Medical Care*, Vol. VI, No. 3, May-June, 1968.

Ordering such tests imposes upon the doctor's time and brings him little reward other than professional satisfaction. Moreover, there appear to be wide variations in the number of tests actually conducted or ordered by general practitioners. Only about 25 percent of British G.P.s account for 75 percent of requests for diagnostic tests.[50]

Even when G.P.s do order tests or conduct them on their own, such tests are usually done in the presence of an apparent illness — not for preventive reasons. In fact, X-rays conducted by G.P.s are rarely performed as part of a general check-up on an apparently healthy person.[51]

Recall that one of Aneurin Bevan's high hopes for the N.H.S. was that it would allow widespread preventive medical care for the

British population. Bevan hoped that by catching diseases in their early stages, the health service would lead to a general improvement in the health of the community. Yet preventive medical care is precisely the type of care that is slighted in the N.H.S. system.

Chest X-rays are actually an exception to this rule. Several years ago, the government by-passed the normal N.H.S. channels and made chest X-rays available to the public through mobile units. Even so, less than half the population receives a chest X-ray every two years.[52]

For other types of preventive care, the record is fairly dismal. For example, even though G.P.s receive an extra fee for cervical cytology tests (PAP smears), most G.P.s will not provide such tests unless patients insist.[53] The attitude is similar for breast checks. Apparently there is a great deal of deterrence going on. In 1976, only 8 percent of eligible females received PAP smears,[54] and most of these were given to middle and upper-middle class patients. (By contrast, in 1973 almost 46% of American women age 17 or older had been given a PAP test within the previous 12 months.) G.P.s also receive extra payments for certain kinds of vaccinations. But again, it appears that the inducement is small. Over the last decade there has been a general decline in the percentage of children vaccinated against every major childhood disease.[55]

Yet another area where the financial incentives and pressures felt by doctors have had an apparent effect upon behavior is that of home visits. This is one area of British health care that most Americans would tend to find attractive. Home visiting is a dying art in the U.S. health care market. It is still alive in Britain, but it's not entirely well.

Most house calls by British physicians occur "after hours" — at night and on the weekends. Technically, the general practitioner is obliged to treat his patients during these hours — especially if he believes there is a medical need. And most patients will receive a visit if they request one.

As one might imagine, a great many things can happen at night and on the weekends that might motivate a patient to seek medical treatment. And since the service is free, patients have an incentive to use it for even the most minor conditions. So like the office visits during the day, the demand for home visits is potentially quite high relative to the supply.

How is the service rationed? In much the same way as day-time services are rationed — by waiting and by a reduction in the quality of the service rendered. Waiting times are apparently not much longer than they are in a doctor's office, although in some instances patients might wait up to four hours.[56] The waiting is done in the patient's home, however — not in the cold and impersonal atmosphere of the doctor's office. The quality of service rendered, though, is probably well below the quality received during office hours.

The reason? The most important reason is that the person who actually calls upon the patient will not be the family doctor at all. It will be someone else taking the G.P.'s place. Although the G.P. is responsible for the patient's care during these hours, the N.H.S. allows him to hire a surrogate, called a "deputy doctor." That is, he can contract out of his obligation by paying another physician to assume his nightly responsibilities. As a result of this freedom, a rather interesting development has occurred within the socialistic confines of the N.H.S. — a nook has been created in which free enterprise can flourish.

Commercial Emergency Treatment Services is an example. This is a company that offers to handle a doctor's off-hour obligations in return for a fee. The company then hires another doctor — usually a low-paid junior hospital doctor — to handle the evening and weekend business. In effect, the company "rents" the substitute to the G.P.

In many cases the G.P. is charged a flat amount per 1,000 patients on his waiting list. In other cases, the G.P. is charged a fee for each visit undertaken. But in either event, the fee paid by the G.P. is often less than the fee paid to the G.P. by the N.H.S. for after-hours visits. So the family doctor himself can often profit from the arrangement.

In 1973, over 7,000 G.P.s subscribed, at least part-time, to these services. Among doctors working in larger cities, about 70 percent are subscribers.[57] Although the arrangement may be profitable for the G.P., the deputy-doctor, and the company that does the "renting," it is not necessarily profitable for the patient.

One problem is that the deputy doctor has even less incentive to provide quality care than the doctor who hires him. Another problem is that the deputy usually knows nothing whatever of the patient's case history. The upshot is that home visits in Britain are not quite as attractive as at first they might seem. The London *Times* explains why:

> The chances are strong that if you live in a city and call out
> your doctor at night or on weekend, he himself will not come.
> Instead, your emergency call will be probably answered by a
> deputy doctor — someone you have never seen before, who

probably does not live in or know your area; who will not have had a chance to study your medical records; who is already tired by long hours of duty in his likely full-time occupation as a hospital doctor; and whose motive for calling is purely financial.

To most British socialists, anything that smacks of free enterprise is tantamount to "profiteering in sickness." But in the case of deputy doctors, there are some non-ideological complaints that can be leveled. The *Times* reports some tragic, and near tragic, cases:

*In Leeds one weekend, a man called on the deputizing services twice to examine his ailing father-in-law. The first doctor dismissed the illness as a touch of bronchitis. The second doctor was even less helpful, and appeared to be slightly drunk. The father-in-law died within 24 hours.

*In the Midlands, a father of a sick nine-year-old boy requested a night visit. The father told the deputy that his son was allergic to most antibiotics, other than epinutin. The doctor ignored this advice, gave the child a different drug, saying, "This one will put him to sleep," and left. Ten minutes later the child turned blue and began choking. He was rushed to the emergency room and remained in the hospital for several days.

*In London, the father of a twelve-month-old baby called a doctor at 3 a.m. His son had a high temperature and his breathing was short. A foreign doctor arrived 45 minutes later, and the deputy and the family had extreme difficulty communicating. Following a cursory examination, the doctor advised the family to contact their G.P. in the morning and left. "As it turned out, it was not serious, but what if it had been?" the father asked.

The Alternatives Open to Patients

One of the most striking results, then, of "free" general practitioner service is the deterioration in the quality of that service. This result is striking but not surprising. As we saw in Chapter 4, a deterioration of quality almost always accompanies price controls. And the greater the discrepancy between the controlled price and the free market price, the greater the deterioration in quality will tend to be. In British medical care markets that discrepancy is as great as it can be, for the money price has been pushed all the way down to zero.

But suppose a patient wants a higher quality of medical care and is willing to do something about it. Is there anything that he can do? Since patients are free to switch doctors, it might seem that shopping around for a doctor would work. Moreover, since doctors have an incentive to expand their list sizes, it would seem that they also have an incentive to improve the quality of their services in order to attract more patients.

There is some evidence that competition among doctors does affect the quality of service rendered. For example, among British patients who have considered changing doctors (an indication of dissatisfaction), 20 percent say they live in an area where no other doctor is available.[58] Apparently, then, where the G.P. has a local monopoly, the quality of service provided tends to be inferior to the quality of service provided by G.P.s who compete with one another.

In areas that have more than one doctor, however, competition often tends to be minimal. Some doctors adopt a "closed shop" policy and refuse to accept patients who wish to change from another doctor in the area. As one doctor explained it, "We say, 'If you don't like him, you won't like me.' "

It's not difficult to see why some doctors would adopt this attitude. While it's true that an extra patient on the list promises to raise the doctor's income, it is also true that the patient who switches is the very last patient that the doctor will want to have on his list. For the switching patient is likely to be a demanding patient, and a demanding patient is precisely the kind of patient the doctor is not interested in courting.

In addition, British patients themselves seem to be surprisingly unaggressive in this area. Many feel their doctors are overworked and underpaid anyway, and do not wish to antagonize them. A great many apparently do not know that they have the right to switch doctors, and of those that do, many do not know how.[59] In addition, the actual mechanics of the transition may be a deterrent. One doctor reported that it takes four months, on the average, to get a new patient's records through the entrails of the N.H.S.[60]

For all of these reasons, then, there is actually very little switching of doctors — unless the patient is forced to change. In fact, 70 percent of all changes occur either because the patient moves or the doctor retires or dies.[61]

One method by which patients do seek to circumvent their general practitioners, however, is through the increased use of Accident and Emergency departments of hospitals. Over the last two decades, there has been a 57 percent increase in new patients attending these departments. As Table 5-5 shows, while there has been steady growth of new attendances, there has not been much change in total attendances at these departments. This reflects the fact that an increasing number of patients are being discharged on the first visit. This in turn suggests that an increasing number of cases are less urgent and more "trivial." Most researchers believe that this trend reflects a growing desire on the part of patients to bypass the deterrents (such as the appointments system) erected by general practitioners.[62] Other investigators have suggested that the initials A and E signify *anything* and *everything*.[63]

Table 5-5
ACCIDENT AND EMERGENCY DEPARTMENTS, TOTAL AND NEW CASES (ENGLAND, PER THOUSAND POPULATION)

	Attendances of New Cases (Accident and Emergency Department)	Total A and E Attendances
1956	114.6	270.0
1961	137.6	291.0
1966	149.4	295.0
1971	170.8	284.9
1975	180.1	273.9

Source: Arthur Gunawardena and Kenneth Lee, "Access and Efficiency in Medical Care: A Consideration of Accident and Emergency Services," in Keith Barnard and Kenneth Lee, eds., *Conflicts in the National Health Service* (London: Croom Helm, 1977), p. 58.

There is yet a third way in which a patient may seek and receive better medical care — through a private arrangement with the doctor. One method of doing this is perfectly legal; the other is illegal. Both patients and their doctors are free to step outside the N.H.S. and make arrangements in the private marketplace. In this case the patient actually pays for his treatment. There are some penalties, however. As with public education, the N.H.S. offers no tax rebate to those who choose not to use its services. In addition, private patients are denied the right to buy drugs for the nominal fee charged by the N.H.S. Once a patient "goes private," he must pay the full cost of the drugs he uses.

Private medicine in Britain will be examined more fully in Chapter 8. For the moment we simply note that it exists, and that those patients who make private arrangements with their doctors apparently feel that the services rendered are sufficiently superior to the normal G.P. services to warrant paying for them.

A final method of circumventing the normal N.H.S. procedures is through the illegal payment of cash for services rendered. Suppose a patient prefers not to wait three days for an appointment and one or two additional hours in a waiting room. An alternative is to offer an illicit payment for prompt service. Under this type of arrangement, the government is not told of the transaction. Both doctor and patient stand to gain. The doctor gains because the patient remains on his N.H.S. list and, thus, he receives his capitation fee from the government in addition to the payment from his patient.[64] The patient gains because he not only receives prompt (and probably better) service, but he retains the ability to purchase drugs for the nominal charges set by the government.

Arrangements such as these are properly described as a *black market*. And black markets not only exist for the normal service of general practitioners, they also exist for other services as well. Take home visits for example. Instead of being attended by a deputy doctor, the patient might well prefer to have his G.P. make the house call. And, for the proper monetary inducement, such a visit might be arranged.

How extensive are these illicit payments? One of the difficulties with illegal activities is that the practitioners are notoriously uncooperative in surveys and polls. My own "unscientific" sampling of former N.H.S. patients and general practitioners suggests that the practice may be widespread.

Who Receives Care?

We have seen that the most important goal of the founding fathers of the N.H.S. was to make health care available on the basis of need, rather than on the basis of ability to pay. For this reason, many defenders of the N.H.S. claim that the N.H.S. should not be evaluated by the economic criteria ordinarily applied to markets for other goods and services. In health care, they claim, the purpose is different — it is not to achieve economic efficiency, but rather a social ideal.

As Ruth Levitt explains, "the crucial point is that the N.H.S.

apart from providing health care, acts as an instrument for redistributing national income." Moreover, what is true of the N.H.S. is also true of other programs operated by the British welfare state. Levitt continues,

> People consume different amounts of these services according to their needs, but they only contribute through taxation what they are required to from an assessment of their income. In this way, for example, families needing more support from social services, housing and the N.H.S. are not financially penalized in comparison with families who need relatively less of this support. In other words, by removing the barrier of "market forces" from health care and other public services, people are free to consume these services according to their needs.[65]

Are British citizens using the N.H.S. on the basis of medical need? The answer must be a resounding *no*. A recent study of ill health in Britain concluded that only 20 percent of the cases in which British citizens develop symptoms of illness result in a visit to a general practitioner.[66] In the remaining 80 percent of the cases, patients either make some attempt at self care (63%) or do nothing at all (16%).

It might be supposed that visits to the general practitioner represent the most serious episodes (and have the greatest medical need). But this turns out not to be true. We have already seen that many, perhaps even a majority, of G.P. consultations are devoted to trivial cases. Nor do the serious cases necessarily receive priority.

Table 5-6 shows a rather astonishing picture of how health care is actually administered in the N.H.S. In over half of the categories listed, there are more patients with an illness who are *not* receiving medical treatment than the number who are being treated.

More recent studies indicate that things are not improving. Multiple screening tests carried out by the Medical Officers of Health within the local government services imply the following: For every case of diabetes, rheumatism or epilepsy known to a general practitioner, there is another case undiagnosed. For every case of psychiatric illness, bronchitis, blood pressure, glaucoma and urinary infection, there are another five cases undiagnosed. For every known case of anaemia, there are eight cases undiagnosed.[67]

Yet another study of the state of British health suggests that medical need is almost irrelevant. Two researchers compared people

Table 5-6

THE CLINICAL ICEBERG: ENGLAND AND WALES, 1962

		No. of recognized sufferers (000)	Estimated total no. of cases (000)	Cases in which no treatment was being sought (000)
Hypertension	males 45+	170	620	450
	females 45+	500	2,720	2,220
Urinary Infection	females 15+	420	830	410
Glaucoma	aged 45+	60	340	280
Epilepsy		160	280	120
Rheumatoid Arthritis	aged 15+	230	520	290
Psychiatric	males 15+	560	1,200	640
Disorders	females 15+	1,290	2,120	830
Diabetes mellitus		290	600	310
Bronchitis	males 45-64	500	980	480
	females 45-64	390	500	110

Source: J.M. Last, "The Clinical Iceberg: England and Wales, 1962," *Lancet,* 1963, II, p. 28.

who, over a ten year period, never saw their doctor with patients who had about an average number of visits. The conclusion: there was little obvious medical difference between the two groups.[68]

So who is it that is actually seeing the doctor? As we saw, Levitt assumed that free medical care would primarily benefit those with low incomes. A number of health economists have reached the same conclusion.[69] The argument is that waiting time in the N.H.S. acts as a deterent to potential patients. And since the time of the high-income worker commands a higher market price than the time of the low-income worker, waiting will be more costly to the former than the latter. As a result, "free" medical care should redistribute consumption from the rich to the poor.

A superficial look at the evidence tends to bear out the argument. As Table 5-7 shows, average visits to a physician vary inversely with social class. In general, the lower a worker's income, the more likely he is to see a general practitioner in any one year. Similar results have been recorded in the United States subsequent to the introduction of Medicaid.[70]

One of the problems with the statistics in Table 5-7 is that they conceal too much. They only tell us how many visits to a physician were made. They do not tell us what happened during the visits. More

Table 5-7

UTILIZATION OF GENERAL PRACTITIONER SERVICES
BY SOCIAL CLASS

Type of Employment	Number of Consultations Per Year
Professionals, employers, and managers	3.4
Intermediate and junior non-manual	3.7
Skilled manual and self-employed non-professional	3.8
Semi-skilled and unskilled manual	4.2

Source: *General Household Survey* (London: Her Majesty's Stationery Office, 1972).

careful studies have inquired into what transpired at the doctor's office, and these studies reveal a very different picture. There is evidence, for example, that "working-class" consultations are more frequently for non-medical reasons than the consultations of "middle-class" patients.[71] There is also evidence that the quality of treatment of illness varies by social class.

One indicator of the quality of service received is the amount of time the doctor actually spends with each patient. A 1973 study, for example, revealed that G.P.s spend about 6.1 minutes on the average with professional patients, and only 4.4 minutes with patients who were manual laborers.[72] A 1976 study reported comparable results — 6.2 minutes for middle-class patients and 4.7 minutes for working-class patients.[73] If these studies are correct, the picture given by Table 5-7 is completely misleading. It would appear that, in any given year, the time spent in medical consultation rises as a patient's income rises.

Other studies have focused on the type of care received by patients who are deemed to "need" care. The method used here is to isolate a particular need for a type of medical treatment, and then see how many patients (in each social class) receive treatment among those who are in need. A 1970 study, for example, found that the "use-to-need" ratios were invariably higher the higher the patient's socioeconomic status in seven separate categories: mass radiography, cervical screening, pregnancy and infant care, dental treatment, breast operations and hospital referrals.[74] More recent studies arrive at similar findings.[75,76]

Not only is inequality widespread within the N.H.S., its existence is so generally accepted that it has assumed the status of a social law. The law, termed the *Inverse Care Law,* was coined several years ago by British general practitioner Julian Hart.[77] According to one version of it, the law states: "the availability of good medical care tends to vary inversely with the need for it in the population served."[78]

In Table 5-8, morbidity statistics for British male workers are broken down by social class. As the table shows, the incidence of illness is considerably greater among the lower classes than it is among middle and upper-middle classes for every category of illness. Yet we have seen that, in general, lower-class patients spend less time with general practitioners and probably receive an inferior quality of care for time they do spend with the doctor. This socioeconomic inequality, then, is an example of the Inverse Care Law.

Table 5-8

VARIATIONS IN THE AVERAGE RATE OF SICKNESS CAUSING LIMITED LONG-STANDING ILLNESS BY SOCIO-ECONOMIC GROUP (MALES ONLY) ENGLAND AND WALES, 1971

Condition	Average rate per 1,000	Professional, employers and managers	Intermediate and junior non-manual	Skilled manual	Semi-skilled and unskilled manual
Mental disorders	11.0	59	65	95	175
Diseases of nervous system	8.7	75	87	79	156
Diseases of eye	7.3	97	112	77	105
Diseases of ear	7.7	56	70	110	142
Heart disease	24.4	83	91	85	141
Other circulatory diseases	10.5	85	70	86	150
Bronchitis	16.9	47	69	106	167
Other low respiratory diseases	13.5	78	96	93	141
Diseases of digestive system	11.4	71	78	101	148
Arthritis and rheumatism	27.5	73	90	79	161
Other diseases of musculoskeletal system	9.3	76	101	99	122
Fractures, etc.	6.3	67	57	105	170
Other injuries	9.5	59	102	100	146

Source: *The General Household Survey — Introductory Report* (London: Her Majesty's Stationery Office, 1973), Tables 8.13 and 8.36.

While the Inverse Care Law is generally acknowledged, there seems to be a great deal of uncertainty about *why* it works. As we saw above, a number of economists expected that rationing-by-waiting in British health care markets would benefit low-income groups relative to high-income groups. What went wrong?

Some partial answers have been provided by Julian LeGrand, Professor of Economics at the University of Sussex.[79] LeGrand argues that there is a fundamental defect in the argument that the poor will be willing to wait longer because they place a lower economic value on their time. The middle-class worker, he points out, is not likely to lose any salary because of a doctor's visit. These workers are generally paid monthly, and absences for doctor's visits are often excused. By contrast, the worker who is paid by the day or the hour is likely to face a real loss of income.

In addition, higher-income patients are more likely to have telephones so that appointments may be easily arranged. Getting to the doctor's office is also easier — higher-income patients are more likely to have cars and thus be less reliant on public transportation. Higher-income groups may also place a higher value on medical services because they are more aware of their potential benefits.

LeGrand also makes a point that has been emphasized by others: doctors may be naturally prone to give better care to members of their own social class. Such factors as a patient's "education, class, manners and sheer persistence will play a significant part" in determining what kind of care he or she receives.[80] One study drew the following conclusion:

> General practitioners knew more about the domestic situation of their middle-class patients, although working-class patients had been with them for longer. Middle-class patients discussed more problems and spent longer in conversation with the doctor. They may also ask more questions and give more information.[81]

LeGrand cites one other factor: the areas where middle-class patients live have more doctors than the areas inhabited by lower-class patients. This factor may be the most important of all. In fact, the original formulation of the Inverse Care Law stated: the least health care is given to *areas* which need it most.[82]

Regional variations in the amount spent on general practice are depicted in Table 5-9. As the table shows, the variation can be considerable. Citizens of Trent, Mersey and Northwestern, for example, receive about 80 percent of the per capita expenditure on G.P. services provided to the residents of N.W. Thames. In addition, N.W. Thames has 20 percent more doctors per capita than the other three regions. If anything, these figures tend to *understate* the problem. For variations from locality to locality within regions tend to be more extreme than the average from region to region.

Table 5-9

GENERAL PRACTITIONERS AND CURRENT SPENDING ON GENERAL MEDICAL SERVICES BY HEALTH REGION

HEALTH REGION	G.P.s PER 10,000 POPULATION. (1977)	PER CAPITA SPENDING (1976)
Northern	4.6	£6.06
Yorkshire	4.7	5.95
Trent	4.5	5.86
East Anglia	4.9	6.38
N.W. Thames	5.5	7.31
N.E. Thames	5.1	5.42
S.E. Thames	5.0	6.24
S.W. Thames	5.2	6.15
Wessex	5.0	6.16
Oxford	4.7	6.24
Southwestern	5.2	6.42
West Midlands	4.6	5.99
Mersey	4.6	5.84
North Western	4.6	5.76

Source: Department of Health and Social Security, *Health and Personal Social Services Statistics for England* (London: Her Majesty's Stationery Office, 1977), Tables 1.3 and 2.7, pp. 15 and 22.
Royal Commission on the National Health Service Report (Merrison Report) (London: Her Majesty's Stationery Office, 1979), Table 14.3, p. 213.

Just how extreme the variations are was investigated by the (London) *Times* a few years ago. In order to test the Inverse Care Law, the *Times* reporters chose to compare differences in the quality of care in various suburbs of Newcastle, a city with few urban problems. As the *Times* explained, "If the Inverse Care Law applies in Newcastle, it is likely to be even more valid elsewhere." Here are some of the findings:

We found considerable evidence to support [the law]. Good family doctors, for example, were far more readily available in stable middle-class suburbs like Jesmond than in Newcastle's working-class West End. Yet on almost every index of health and hygiene, the West End has worse problems. Its infant mortality rate is twice as high. Almost half its children in infant and junior schools were found to be infected with body lice, compared with only one in 14 in Jesmond![83]

The West End of Newcastle is by no means the worst case. The quality of health care delivered in places like the mining areas of South Wales is probably far inferior to the quality of care administered anywhere in Newcastle.

In general, those areas with the greatest health needs tend not only to receive the least care, they also tend to have the fewest doctors. The N.H.S. bureaucracy has long been aware of this problem, and those areas where the shortage of general practitioners is critical are officially labeled "under-doctored."

As we have seen, doctors have some financial inducement to locate in those areas. But, not surprisingly, general practitioners prefer to practice in areas where they prefer to live. The financial inducement to locate in undesirable areas has apparently not been sufficient. Between 1965 and 1975, the percentage of N.H.S. patients living in "under-doctored" areas grew from 17 percent to 35 percent.[84] Only in recent years has this trend shown any sign of reversing itself.

Economic Efficiency in General Practice

Is the market for the services of general practitioners an efficient one? Evidence suggests that it is not. Most observers agree that much of the work being done in hospitals could be performed more efficiently by G.P.s practicing on their own or in community health centers. When the great majority of G.P.s have few medical instruments beyond stethoscopes and blood-pressure cuffs, and must send their patients to hospitals for even chest X-rays and simple blood-tests,[85] avoidable costs are being imposed — not only on the N.H.S., but on patients as well. Similarly, the practice of allowing emergency-room doctors and hospital specialists to act as surrogate G.P.s reflects the perverse incentives created by the N.H.S., and has little effect on cost-minimizing the delivery of medical care.

More serious still, however, is the way in which the G.P.'s time is allocated. Comparisons between general practice in Britain and in the United States suggest that there is a great deal of economic waste in British primary medical care. Many expatriate British G.P.s practicing in the U.S. have noted a similarity between the mechanical, revolving-door type of treatment meted out to Medicaid and Medicare patients here, and the conditions of general practice back home. On the other hand, where U.S. patients pay their own bills, or the bulk of them, the differences between the two countries are striking. On the average, Americans see a G.P. about once every year,[86] while

British patients make about four G.P. visits annually.[87] Yet when American patients do see their family doctor, they spend about two and one-half times as much time with him as British patients spend with their doctors. A reasonable inference, then, is that if British patients were paying for the cost of G.P. services out of their own pockets, they would make fewer trips to doctors' offices and would expect a higher quality of services on those trips they did make. Evidence from other countries confirms the inference. Even when user fees are only nominal, they appear to affect behavior:

> A 12 kroner standard fee for a doctor's visit in Sweden ... would not pay for a haircut. In Germany, 2.50DM for medicines is not much more than the cost of a packet of cigarettes (but in New Zealand, the flat rate for medicines is set at two packets of cigarettes). For the most part it can be said that when user charges are levied, they are typically not really a barrier for "essential" care but act to dissuade or ration treatments which are considered to be "non-essential."[88]

The number of home visits made by British doctors is another example. While exact statistics are not available, I would guess that British G.P.s may make as many as 1.75 million house calls annually at a total cost (to the N.H.S.) which may run as high as $60 million.[89] In the U.S., neither law nor custom prevents home visits by general practitioners; and, if the price were right, no doubt most G.P.s would offer the service. Yet when patients are paying their own bills, it appears that the service is simply not worth the cost. It's more economical to have the patient go to the doctor. That is probably the major reason why home visits in the U.S. are rare and the practice is now predicted to be moving toward extinction.[90]

Why are things so different in Britain? The difference cannot be explained solely by the fact that the two economies are different. A recent study comparing G.P. practice in Iowa and Northwestern England, each a relatively isolated area, confirmed that a larger proportion of home visits occurs in Britain.[91] Again, it is probably reasonable to infer that the British demand for home visits would be greatly diminished if patients were individually footing the bill.

General practice in Britain, then, seems to be characterized by a lot of waste and inefficiency. Because G.P. services are made free to the user at the time they are consumed, the average British patient simply isn't getting his money's worth for the tax dollars he pays to finance these services. What's more, the average patient ends up paying more (in tax dollars) for many services than those services are really worth to him. At the same time, services he would like to have and would be willing to pay for are simply not being made available.

More generally, British general practice appears to be inefficient for another reason: there are too many general practitioners relative to specialists in the N.H.S. In the United States, only about 17 percent of all physicians are general practitioners. In Britain, the percentage of general practitioners is about three times as high.[92] While G.P. services are important in both countries, the majority of G.P. visits pertain to conditions which are medically trivial. Britain, however, clearly devotes a far greater proportion of its resources to this kind of care. In return, British patients pay a price. To see what kind of price they pay, we need to turn to the hospital sector.

Footnotes

1. "Equal Care, The Decline of a Social Ideal," (London) *Times,* May 13, 1973.
2. J. Ashford and N.G. Pearson, "Who Uses Health Services and Why?" *Journal of the Royal Statistical Society,* 133, 3, Series A, 1970.
3. Economic Models, Ltd., *The British Health Care System* (Chicago: American Medical Association, 1976), p. 99.
4. Department of Health and Social Security, *Health and Personal Social Services Statistics for England,* 1977 (London: Department of Health and Social Security, 1977), Table 3.29, p. 61 and Table 3.32, p. 64.
5. Economic Models, Ltd., *The British Health Care System,* p. 78. Part of the reason for the decline appears to have been a spectacular misjudgment on the part of health planners. In 1955, a government committee recommended that medical school admissions be cut by 10 percent. In projecting the need for G.P.s, the committee estimated that the British population would grow at a rate of 4.5 percent between 1955 and 1971. The actual growth rate was nearly double that figure. See "The Decline of a Social Ideal," (London) *Times.*
6. Ruth Levitt, *The Reorganized National Health Service* (London: Croom Helm, Ltd., 1976), p. 95.
7. Cartwright, *Patients and their Doctors,* p. 48.
8. Michael H. Cooper, *Rationing Health Care* (New York: Halsted Press, 1975), pp. 12-13.
9. *Ibid,* p. 13.
10. *Ibid,* p. 14.
11. *Ibid,* pp. 16 and 17.
12. *Ibid,* pp. 16-18. Sickness due to influenza has been excluded from these statistics because epidemics tend to obscure the underlying trend.
13. Organization for Economic Cooperation and Development, *Public Expenditure on Health* (Paris: OECD, 1977), p. 52, n. 25.
14. D.F. Crombie, "Morbidity Statistics from General Practice," in *Risks and Uncertainty in Medical Care* (London: Office of Health Economics, 1974).
15. There was an increase in the reported incidence of every non-serious ailment except skin and stomach disorders.
16. Enoch Powell, *Medicine and Politics: 1975 and After* (New York: Pitman, 1976), p. 16.
17. Data obtained from the National Center for Health Statistics, U.S. Department of Health, Education and Welfare.
18. Mary-Ann Rozbicki, *Rationing British Health Care: The Cost/Benefit Approach,* Executive Seminar in National and International Affairs, U.S. Department of State, April, 1978, p. 8.
19. Anthony J. Culyer, *Need and the National Health Service* (Totowa, New Jersey: Rowman and Littlefield, 1976), p. 84.
20. David Cunningham, "How I Twice Survived Socialized Medicine," *Private Practice,* May, 1978, p. 101.
21. D. Mechanic, "General Practice in England and Wales: Results from a Survey of a National Sample of General Practitioners," *Medical Care,* Vol. 6, No. 3, May-June, 1968.
22. Cartwright, *Patients and Their Doctors,* p. 40.
23. Economic Models, Ltd., *The British National Health Care System,* p. 85.
24. Derrick Henderson, "The British Triangle," *Private Practice,* April, 1978, p. 57.
25. *Ibid,* pp. 56-57.
26. Calculated at a Conversion rate of $2 = £1. See Economic Models, Ltd., *The British Health Care System,* p. 97, Table 1.
27. *Ibid.*
28. Mechanic, "General Practice in England and Wales."
29. The N.H.S. places a maximum of 3,500 on list sizes, however.
30. Powell, *Medicine and Politics,* pp. 32-33.
31. Brian Abel-Smith, *Value for Money in Health Services* (New York: St. Martin's Press,

1976), p. 54. The difference between American and British malpractice law is discussed more fully in Chapter 6.

32. Cooper, *Rationing Health Care*, p. 53.
33. *Ibid.*
34. Cartwright, *Patients and their Doctors.*
35. Cooper, *Rationing Health Care*, p. 54.
36. It appears, however, that the reduction in waiting time has been minimal. See A. Cartwright and R. Anderson, *Patients and the Doctors*, 1977, Institute for Social Studies in Medical Care, Royal College of General Practitioners, Occasion Paper No. 8, 1979.
37. Cooper, *Rationing Health Care*, p. 54.
38. J.M. Last, "Objective Measurement of Quality in General Practice," *Supplement to the Annals of G.P.* (Australia), Vol. 12, No. 2, 1967.
39. R. Scott and M. Gilmore, "The Edinburgh Hospitals," in G. McLaughland (ed.) *Problems and Progress in Medical Care* (Oxford: Oxford University Press, 1966).
40. G. Forsyth and R.F.L. Logan, *Gateway or Dividing Line* (Oxford: Nuffield Provincial Hospitals Trust, 1968).
41. Cooper, *Rationing Health Care*, p. 102.
42. Donald Gould, "Delivering Health Care Wisely and Well," *New Scientist*, Vol. 74, April 7, 1977, p. 16.
43. Cooper, *Rationing Health Care*, p. 102.
44. "Equal Care, the Decline of a Social Ideal," (London) *Times*, p. 34.
45. Henderson, "The British Triangle," pp. 57-58.
46. Powell, *Medicine and Politics*, p. 33.
47. Levitt, *The Reorganized National Health Service*, p. 95.
48. D. Irvine and M. Jeffreys, "BMA Planning Unit Survey of General Practice," *British Medical Journal*, 4, (1971), 535.
49. "Equal Care, the Decline of a Social Ideal," (London) *Times*, p. 33.
50. Levitt, *The Reorganized National Health Service*, p. 97.
51. Cartwright, *Patients and Their Doctors*, pp. 80-81.
52. *Ibid*, p. 78.
53. Rozbicki, *Rationing British Health Care*, p. 8.
54. *Health and Personal Social Services Statistics for England*, pp. 14 and 165.
55. *Ibid*, p. 164
56. "Equal Care: The Decline of a Social Ideal," (London) *Times*. Most of the following analysis has been adapted from the report in the *Times*.
57. *Ibid.*
58. Cartwright, *Patients and Their Doctors*, p. 22.
59. *Ibid.*
60. "Equal Care: The Decline of a Social Ideal," (London) *Times*, p. 33.
61. Cartwright, *Patients and Their Doctors*, p. 21.
62. Cooper, *Rationing Health Care*, p. 54.
63. Arthur Gunawardena and Kenneth Lee, "Access and Efficiency in Medical Care: A Consideration of Accident and Emergency Service," in Keith Barnard and Kenneth Lee, eds., *Conflicts in the National Health Service* (London: Croom Helm, 1977), p. 58.
64. In addition, the payment is undoubtedly overlooked when the doctor's income tax statement is filed.
65. Levitt, *The Reorganized National Health Service*, p. 215.
66. Cooper, *Rationing Health Care*, p. 12.
67. *Ibid*, p. 13.
68. N. Kessel and M. Sheppard, "The Health Attitudes of People Who Seldom Consult a Doctor," *Medical Care*, Vol. 3, No. 6, 1965.
69. See D. Nichols, E. Smolensky and T.N. Tideman, "Discrimination by Waiting Time in Merit Goods," *American Economic Review*, Vol. 63, 1971; and E. Smolensky, T.N. Tide-

man and D. Nichols, "Waiting Time as a Congestion Charge," in S. Mushkin (ed.) *Public Prices for Public Products* (Washington, D.C.: Urban Institute, 1972).

70. The effects of Medicaid in the U.S. are indicated by the following:
    Number of visits per person per year:

	"Poor"	"Non-Poor"
1964	4.3	4.6
1973	5.6	4.9

    Percent with no physician visits in past two years:

1964	27.7	17.7
1973	17.2	13.4

    See OECD, *Public Expenditures on Health*, pp. 46-47.

71. Cooper, *Rationing Health Care*, p. 15.

72. I. Buchan and I. Richardson, *Time Study of Consultations in General Practice,* Scottish Health Service Studies, no. 27, Scottish Home and Health Department (Edinburgh: Her Majesty's Stationery Office, 1973).

73. A. Cartwright and M. O'Brien, "Social Class Variations in Health Care and the Nature of General Practice Consultations," in M. Stacey, ed., *The Sociology of the National Health Service*, Sociological Review Monograph, no. 22 (Keele: University Press, 1976).

74. M. R. Alderson, "Social Class and the Health Service," *The Medical Officer*, 124 (1970), 52.

75. D. P. Forster, "Social Class Differences in Sickness and General Practitioner Consultations," *Health Trends*, 8 (1976), 29-32.

76. Cartwright and O'Brien, "Social Class Variations in Health Care," p. 93.

77. "Equal Care," (London) *Times*, p. 37.

78. Kenneth Lee, "Public Expenditure, Planning and Local Democracy," in Barnard and Lee, *Conflicts in the National Health Service*, p. 223.

79. Julian LeGrand, "The Distribution of Public Expenditure: The Case of Health Care," *Economica*, vol. 45, No. 178, May, 1978, pp. 137-138.

80. Cooper, *Rationing Health Care*, p. 20.

81. Cartwright and O'Brien, "Social Class Variations in Health Care," p. 94.

82. "Equal Care," (London) *Times*, p. 33.

83. *Ibid.*

84. *Ibid.*

85. Harry Swartz, "The Infirmity of British Medicine," in Emmett Tyrrell, Jr., ed., *The Future That Doesn't Work: Social Democracy's Failures in Britain* (New York: Doubleday, 1977), p. 29.

86. Data obtained from the National Center for Health Statistics, U.S. Department of Health, Education and Welfare.

87. Cooper, *Rationing Health Care*, p. 8.

88. OECD, *Public Expenditure on Health*, p. 45.

89. These estimates are based on the conjectures contained in *The British Health Care System*, Table 11, p. 97.

90. Derek Robinson, "Primary Medical Practice in the United Kingdom and the United States," *New England Journal of Medicine*, Vol. 297, No. 4, July 28, 1977, p. 190.

91. G.N. Marsh, R.B. Wallace and J. Whewell, "Anglo-American Contrasts in General Practice," *British Medical Journal*, 2, 1976.

92. See *Health and Personal Social Services Statistics,* pp. 28-29.

Chapter 6
Rationing: The Hospital Sector

The British health care system is basically a hospital-based system. Hospitals absorb about two-thirds of the N.H.S. budget and, despite the recent emergence of community health centers, the hospitals' share of N.H.S. spending seems unlikely to decline in the near future.[1]

In any given year, about 24 percent of the population attends hospitals as out-patients, and another 10 percent are admitted as in-patients.[2] Those who do attend hospitals as out-patients average about 2.7 attendances per year. So on the average, individuals attend hospitals as out-patients about once every one and one-half years. Over a lifetime, the average British citizen can expect to be an in-patient in a hospital about eight times and spend about three and one-half weeks in the hospital for each episode.[3]

The central problem of the hospital sector is the same problem faced by general practitioners — with medical services free to the patient at the time they are consumed, the quantity of services demanded far exceeds the quantity supplied. In the hospital sector, however, the rationing problem is far greater, and the effects on health far more serious, than the rationing problem encountered by general practitioners.

The Waiting Lists

By the end of the first year of operation of the N.H.S., it was painfully obvious that the demand for hospital services far exceeded the supply. In December of 1949, for example, 460,000 people were on waiting lists to get into British hospitals. What was *not* obvious, at least to the N.H.S. administrators at that time, was that the waiting lists were a permanent feature of the British health care system. Twenty years later, in December of 1969, the number of people on waiting lists stood at 561,000, and by 1979 they totaled about 750,000.

The lion's share of the list consists of people waiting for surgery. In 1976, for example, about 82 percent of those waiting were surgical cases.[4] On the average, patients can expect to wait a little over three months before they are admitted.[5] There are a great many patients, however, who far exceed the average. For example, it is apparently not uncommon for patients to wait up to three years for simple ear, nose and throat operations. Patients often wait two to three years for gall bladder operations, and an elderly arthritic can wait up to two years for a hip replacement.[6] A survey taken in 1975 found that in six major surgical specialties, 37 percent of the patients had been waiting for longer than a year, nearly 20 percent for longer than two years, and some for longer than four years.[7]

A rather extreme example of waiting conditions was recently brought to light by Dr. John Cozens-Hardy, one of Britain's leading orthopedic surgeons. The surgeon went so far as to hire a public hall to explain to his patients why they had to spend years "imprisoned by constant pain." At the present rate, he told them, it would take 36 years to clear the 127 people on his waiting list. The delay, he said, was due to a chronic shortage of beds, operating rooms and trained medical staff. As the surgeon explained to reporters after the meeting:

> The 127 I have invited . . . suffer pain 24 hours a day. I am paid to help these people, but I am denied the opportunity. They have paid, through their contributions and taxes, for that help. When this ever-worsening situation goes on year after year, one reaches the point where one either resigns, commits suicide, or screams. I have decided to scream.[8]

If there are those who considerably exceed the average waiting time, there must be plenty of people who gain hospital admission rather promptly. So what determines who receives treatment quickly and who waits? *In theory,* the determination is based on medical need.

Patients are generally classified into one of three groups: "emergency" (critical), "urgent", and "non-urgent". Emergency patients have top priority and are treated immediately. Urgent cases receive next priority, followed by non-urgent. Patients in need of orthopedic or gall bladder surgery, or nose, eye and throat operations are generally considered to be non-urgent patients — they may be living in pain, but their conditions are not life-threatening.

Until very recently, Ministers of Health routinely defended the N.H.S. waiting lists by stating that all patients on waiting lists were non-urgent cases. In other words, patients may suffer some inconvenience, but no one's life is threatened by waiting.

That claim is no longer plausible. In 1977, David Ennals, Secretary of State for Social Services, admitted that 40,000 urgent cases were on waiting lists.[9] Moreover, as early as 1971, a survey of waiting lists by the Department of Health and Social Security found cases of "urgent" patients who had waited for more than a year.[10]

In addition, the British Press and medical journals these days are filled with horror stories confirming the hazardous effects of waiting: an open-heart operation is twice postponed for a Welsh woman because there is no bed for her in the intensive care unit. She dies at home shortly thereafter.[11] A sixty-six year old man suffers a stroke but is denied admission to the nearest hospital because no one over sixty-five is supposed to be treated there.[12] One hospital actually had twenty *unconscious* patients on its admissions waiting list, and "sent a trained health visitor round to assess the priority of these cases, presumedly to see who was the most unconscious."[13]

One of the difficulties in assessing the seriousness of the waiting lists is that the terms "emergency," "urgent," and "non-urgent" do not have objective or operational definitions. As former Minister of Health Enoch Powell has pointed out, in assigning these terms to specific cases, doctors are naturally influenced by the availability of medical treatment.[14] If the capacity of the hospital is expanded, more urgent cases might be reclassified as "emergency," and more non-urgent cases might be classified as "urgent." The reverse would be true if the hospital's capacity to treat patients is diminished.

In any event, many patients classified as urgent and waiting for entry into British hospitals are risking their lives and health by simply having to wait. Dr. Nigel Harris, honorary secretary of the Hospital Consultants and Specialists Association, explains why:

> A patient waiting for surgery to improve the blood flow in the legs may instead have to have an amputation because of irreversible changes in the tissues; a cancer which could have been removed when first suspected may have advanced so that only palliative treatment is possible; a rheumatoid joint may have so deteriorated that the success rate of the operation is much reduced. Some patients awaiting cardiac surgery die of their disease before they can be treated.[15]

Another difficulty in assessing the seriousness of waiting lists is that the British government has been largely uninterested in discovering what costs are imposed upon patients who are on these lists. It is a remarkable fact that in the first 30 years since the inception of the N.H.S., not a single survey was taken of waiting patients to discover what costs were imposed upon them by the system of rationing by waiting.[16]

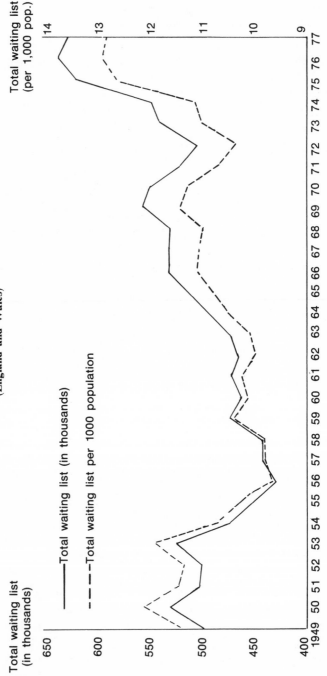

Figure 6-1

HOSPITAL WAITING LISTS, 1949-1977

(England and Wales)

Source: Michael Cooper, *Rationing Health Care* (New York: Halsted Press, 1975), Table 4, p. 23, and Central Statistical Office, *Annual Abstract of Statistics*, 1979 (London: Her Majesty's Stationery Office, 1978), Table 3.41, p. 80.

The Demand For Hospital Services

Throughout most of the history of the N.H.S., the number of people on hospital waiting lists has been regarded as a measure of "excess demand." That is, the number of people waiting to gain hospital admission was regarded as that part of the total demand for hospital services that could not be immediately satisfied. A consequence of this attitude was that a succession of Ministers of Health tried mightily to "get the waiting lists down." Yet, as Enoch Powell has observed, this "is an activity about as hopeful as filling a sieve."[17]

Between 1949 and 1971 there was about a 100 percent increase in the annual patient case load handled by British hospitals.[18] Yet as Figure 6-1 shows, despite this increase in case load, both the number of people on hospital waiting lists and the ratio of those waiting to the total population have actually increased. Why? The major reason is that the total hospital waiting list does not really reflect the excess demand for hospital services. This is because of the activities of both doctors and patients. In general, a patient joins a waiting list after obtaining the advice and consent of a hospital doctor. Moreover, a patient sees the doctor only after a referral from a general practitioner or the hospital's out-patient department.

There is evidence that the referral practices of general practitioners and the attitudes of hospital doctors are heavily influenced by the capacity of the system to treat new patients. As Michael Cooper puts it, "doctors appear to be assessing the need for referrals and admissions as a simple function of current provision levels."[19] In other words, if the supply of hospital services is increased, and the total waiting list decreased, doctors simply reevaluate their patients' needs in the light of these circumstances. They then proceed to increase referrals and, consequently, the number of patients officially awaiting admission.[20]

Perhaps an equally important reason why the waiting lists do not accurately reflect the full extent of unsatisfied demand is that the waiting list *itself* acts as a "price." In a private market place, money prices ration limited quantities of goods and services among the many people who would like to consume them. In the N.H.S., where money prices have been abolished, the waiting list serves the same function.

As we saw in Chapter 4, rationing by waiting is simply another form of rationing. In gasoline markets in the United States in 1973 and 1979, the length of the waiting line imposed a cost on those who wanted gasoline. Those car owners who actually got gasoline were the ones who were willing to pay the "price" of waiting. In a similar way, "in the hospital service probably the most pervasive, certainly the most palpable, form of rationing is the waiting list."[21]

Not only does the waiting list act as a general "price" for hospital services, specific lists for specific surgeons act as differential prices for differences in experience and skill. The waiting lists of hospital consultants in the same department of a hospital can differ greatly in length. As Powell explains it, "there has to be some differential rationing for different qualities of an article; and if not price, then, for example time: better surgeon, longer wait, and vice versa."[22]

The waiting list, then, simply tells us how many potential patients are willing to pay the "price" of waiting. Those who are unwilling to pay this price may seek private medical care, or go without medical care altogether. But if the "price" is lowered, say, because the list or the average waiting time is shortened, we would expect more people to join the queue.

This is precisely the behavioral response that economic studies have confirmed. An early study by Harvard economist Martin Feldstein of 177 large, acute hospitals found that both hospital admissions and average length of stay in hospitals increased with bed availability. Moreover, Feldstein could discover no indication of a bed provision level which would have fully satiated the demand for hospital services.[23] Similar conclusions were reached by two more recent economic studies conducted by Culyer and Cullis.[24]

The evidence, then, suggests that not only are waiting lists not an indicator of excess demand, but that the true demand for hospital services is virtually infinite. The general principle is expressed by *Parkinson's law of hospital beds,* which asserts that "the number of patients always tends to equality with the number of beds for them to lie in."[25]

On the whole, the relationship of the demand for hospital services to the hospital waiting list has been ably summarized by Enoch Powell:

> Generally, the waiting list can be viewed as a kind of iceberg: the significant part is that below the surface — the patients who are not on the list at all, either because they are not accepted on the grounds that the list is too long already or because they take a look at the queue and go away. Naturally, no one knows how many there are. Indeed, the very question is rather absurd, as it implies some natural, inherent limitation of demand. But the part of the iceberg above the water

is doing its work, directly as well as indirectly, by attrition as well as by deterrence.

It might be thought macabre to observe that if people are on a waiting list long enough, they will die — usually for some cause other than that for which they joined the queue. Short of dying, however, they frequently get bored or better, and vanish. Here again, time on the waiting list is a communtation not only for money — measurable by the cost of private treatment with less or no delay — but also for the other good things of life.[26]

As is the case with the demand for general practitioner services, the demand for hospital services includes the serious as well as the trivial. And, in theory, hospital care is supposed to be meted out on the basis of medical need, with the most serious conditions receiving priority over the less serious.

There is considerable evidence, however, that the practical, day-to-day operations of the hospital sector often stray wide of the theoretical mark. As we saw in Chapter 5, a great many British citizens with serious medical conditions are not seeing a doctor at all. Moreover, of those people on hospital waiting lists, there is substantial evidence that those with the most serious conditions are not necessarily at the top of the list.

At the same time that many "urgent" cases go untreated, it appears that many patients near the top of some hospital lists turn down treatment for other activities. As Enoch Powell has observed:

It is an interesting phenomenon of the waiting lists for in-patient treatment that at the holiday season and around Christmas time it may be necessary to go quite far down a lengthy waiting list to get patients willing to accept the long-awaited treatment in sufficient numbers to keep even the temporarily reduced hospital resources fully employed.[27]

One reason why medical treatment is not necessarily administered in accordance with the severity of medical need is that there appears to be no nationally uniform standard for determining waiting list priorities; or, for that matter, for determining who should be on the waiting list at all. Studies show that wide variations exist in general practitioner referral rates,[28] in admission rates among hospital doctors,[29] and in the length of the waiting lists from region to region.[30] Moreover, in a survey of the admissions policies of 92 British hospitals, 45 percent reported that there was no accepted criteria for determining who should be included on the waiting list.[31]

Another reason why medical treatment is not necessarily administered in accordance with medical need is that there is no mechanism for equalizing the backlog of serious cases across different areas of the country. The number of persons waiting for a heart operation, for example, is six times greater in London than in Merseyside.[32]

There is no doubt that other factors are also important determinants of how long a patient waits to gain admission to a hospital — the patient's persistence, general educational level and social class, or the existence of black market arrangements. But one factor that is clearly important in determining who receives treatment and how quickly treatment is administered is the conscious decision on the part of the government and the N.H.S. administrators to make more, or less, of certain types of hospital services available.

The Supply of Hospital Care

In a socialized medical scheme, two important political decisions must be made concerning the supply of medical services: (1) *how much* medical care should be supplied; and (2) *what kind* of medical care should be supplied?

We have already seen how the first of these questions has been answered in the hospital sector. Out of a relatively meager N.H.S. budget, roughly two-thirds has been allocated to hospitals. Moreover, the quantity of services provided is far below what the British public demands in the absence of money prices. What is most striking, and to most American observers even alarming, about the British health care system, however, is the way in which the second question has been answered.

In deciding what types of hospital services to provide, the British system reveals two marked preferences: (1) a preference for current expenditure over capital expenditure; and (2) a preference for routine and less expensive treatment over newer, more expensive, and more potent techniques made available by modern medical science.

Capital expenditure refers to expenditures on buildings and expensive equipment. *Current expenditure* refers to expenditures on wages and salaries, maintenance and other day-to-day expenses. Capital expenditure is an investment. The benefits of a new building or a new piece of diagnostic equipment are not fully realized in the current period. These benefits will be extended over many years. So capital expenditures made today are largely an investment in medical benefits which will be realized in the future. By contrast, current expenditures create benefits which are fully realized in the current period. In choosing between these two types of expenditures, the British have displayed a myopia which often characterizes political decision-making. Their preference: benefits now!

One of the reasons often cited for the creation of the N.H.S. was "the need to modernize and expand Britain's antiquated hospital system."[33] Yet during the first 15 years of operation of the N.H.S., only one new hospital was constructed.[34] Although the next 15 years saw a marked increase in hospital construction (forty new hospitals had been built by 1972), about 50 percent of the hospital beds in Britain today are in buildings that were built before the turn of the century. These are buildings that one observer has described as "obsolete" and "offering facilities in many respects more akin to a railway station than a place for the ailing."[35]

In the early 1970s, plans were made for a substantial increase in hospital construction. But by 1976, political pressures were firmly at work. Declaring that the N.H.S. must "put people before buildings," a 1976 Consultative Document[36] laid down the government's new priorities: capital spending would be cut back from 528 million pounds in 1973/74 to an estimated 424 million pounds in 1975/76, and 304 million pounds in 1979/80. Moreover, the hospital sector was expected to absorb about two-thirds of the projected cut in capital funds available.[37]

Perhaps more revealing than the statistics on hospital construction are the statistics on hospital beds. From 1900 to 1938, the number of hospital beds in England and Wales increased by over 400 percent.[38] Yet there are fewer hospital beds in Britain today than when the N.H.S. was founded![39] As Table 6-1 shows, even in recent years the decline in the number of beds has been steady — in absolute terms, as a percentage of the population, and as a percentage of the number of persons on hospital waiting lists.

One reason why the number of hospital beds has declined, despite the building of new hospitals, is the inordinate number of hospitals and hospital wards that have been closed. Since 1970, 30 hospitals have been closed and another 50 are threatened with closure over the next decade.[40] Such closings are often accompanied by widespread demonstrations and "occupations" in an attempt to prevent the shutdowns. In one instance, patients were even forcibly evacuated from a condemned hospital.[41]

Ironically, while many old hospitals are being forced to close, some new hospitals and hospital wards are standing empty. In 1978,

Table 6-1
HOSPITAL BEDS, 1965-1977[1]

Year	No. of Beds (thousands)	No. of Beds Per 1,000 Population	No. of People on Waiting Lists (thousands)	No. of Beds Per Person Waiting[2]
1965	470	9.9	517	0.91
1966	468	9.8	536	0.87
1967	467	9.7	537	0.87
1968	465	9.6	535	0.86
1969	461	9.5	561	0.82
1970	455	9.3	556	0.82
1971	450	9.2	526	0.86
1972	443	9.0	510	0.87
1973	437	8.9	545	0.80
1974	427	8.7	553	0.77
1975	419	8.5	626	0.67
1976	412	8.4	644	0.64
1977	404	8.2	637	0.63

1. Figures are for December 31 each year and refer to England and Wales.
2. If Scotland and Northern Ireland were included, the ratio would be lower.
Source: *Annual Abstract of Statistics*, 1978 and 1979 (London: Her Majesty's Stationery Office).

new hospitals in Liverpool, Oxford and Sheffield and elsewhere were unable to open because of the lack of staff and money. And a prominent specialist in intensive care recently claimed that the failure to open just one completed unit at the world famous Stoke-Mandeville Hospital is causing 100 to 150 avoidable deaths each year.[42]

While the N.H.S. has skimped on buildings and beds, it has been far less stingy on hiring personnel. Since 1949, the ratio of doctors employed by the N.H.S. to patients has risen from 1:1,435 to 1:1,180.[43] As Table 6-2 shows, most of this improvement is due to the more than doubling of hospital doctors. The table also shows that between 1949 and 1971, there was a 109 percent increase in the nursing staff and a 164 percent increase in the professional and technical staff, while the British population increased by only 11 percent. Indeed, one health expert has observed that the current trends in hospital manpower suggest that by the twenty-first century, half the population will be employed in hospitals.[44]

Not only has the N.H.S. dramatically increased its hospital personnel, but wages and salaries paid to hospital personnel are consuming an ever-increasing share of the current expense budget. In 1968, the weekly earnings of N.H.S. male manual workers were 80 percent of the average earnings of male manual workers outside the

Table 6-2
MANPOWER CHANGES, 1949-1971
(England and Wales)

	Unit	1949	1971	% change
Hospital Service				
Ancillary staff (porters, etc.)	No	157,112	239,770	52.6
Professional and technical	*Wte	13,940	36,817	164.1
Medical staff	*Wte	11,735	23,806	102.9
(consultants)		(3,488)	(8,655)	(148.1)
Dental staff	*Wte	206	753	265.5
Nursing staff	No	137,636	288,065	109.3
Administrative and clerical	No	23,797	47,690	100.4
Regional Board staff	No	1,320	7,243	448.7
Executive Council				
General practitioners				
(all principals)	No	20,400	23,707	16.2
Dentists	No	9,495	10,962	15.5
Ophthalmic medical				
practitioners	No	996	920	7.6
Population	(000)	43,785	48,815	11.5

*Wte — whole time equivalents.
Source: Michael Cooper, *Rationing Health Care* (New York: Halsted Press, 1975),
    Table 12, p. 37.

health service. For women (whose average work week is longer), the figure was 106 percent. By 1975, however, the corresponding percentages had risen to 91 percent for men and 118 percent for women.[45] Moreover, during roughly the same period of time, over 70 percent of each year's increase in hospital spending was attributable to increases in wages and prices alone — that is, over 70 percent of all additional spending consisted of nothing more than paying higher prices for the same services.[46]

Can we conclude that the British have devoted too much of the health service budget to current expenditure and too little to capital expenditure? A conclusion such as this is difficult to make about a system where prices are not allowed to reflect public preferences and values. With health care "free" to the user, there is a shortage in every aspect of hospital service. There are constant complaints both from within and without the health service that there is too little of everything — too few personel, too few beds and too few hospitals.

Another difficulty with drawing firm conclusions in this area is that the hospital sector seems to be plagued by some gross inefficiencies. For example, although there is certainly a bed shortage in the hospital sector, there are more beds per person in Britain than in the

United States.[47] Nonetheless, in the U.S. the average patient spends much less time in the hospital and, as a consequence, a greater percentage of the U.S. population receives hospital treatment each year than in Britain.[48] Were the British hospitals as "efficient" in treating patients as American hospitals apparently are, the British need for hospital beds would be lessened. We will examine this feature of the hospital sector in more detail later.

Despite these difficulties, there are three general observations we can make about capital and current spending in the N.H.S. First, compared to other countries where government ownership of hospitals is widespread, the British devote a small proportion of their budget to capital expenditure.[49] Second, perhaps more than most other industrialized nations, the British have an inordinately obsolete capital stock. Third, there is little indication that the *political will* exists to make any major shift in spending priorities.

Another way in which the N.H.S. has skimped on capital expenditure is the area of new medical technology. The EMI brain scanner is a remarkable machine that has revolutionized the diagnosis of brain disease and brain injuries and, in the process, has saved a great many lives. Its technological cousin, the full-body CAT scanner, goes further by permitting the early detection and successful treatment of such diseases as lung cancer. Ironically, Britain is the country where scanner technology was invented. Yet as late as 1976, there were in all of Britain less than two dozen brain scanners being used.[50] And as late as 1977, Britain was using only four full-body scanners.[51] By contrast, in the United States (with a population about four times that of Britain), there are over 1,000 scanners (over half of which were produced in Britain). Moreover, recent improvements in this area are largely due to public — not N.H.S. — decision makers. Of the twenty full body scanners in use in 1979, half were donated to the N.H.S. by individuals and private charitable organizations.[52]

A more flagrant example of premeditated refusal to buy expensive technology lies in the field of renal dialysis. The incidence of treatable chronic renal failure is small in most Western industrialized countries — about 40 to 150 people per million population annually. Yet for those who are afflicted, life-saving treatment is expensive — either a kidney transplant or a renal dialysis machine is needed. Ironically, Britain was also an early pioneer in the development of renal dialysis. But in 1976, the N.H.S. accepted only 15 new patients per million population. That means that up to 8,100 people needlessly died that year because the N.H.S. refused to buy additional dialysis machines![53] The decision in 1978 to purchase 400 additional dialysis machines will put a small dent in this number.

How much does renal treatment cost? British studies estimate that the annual cost of treatment in 1976/77 prices averages about £5,000 (or $10,000).[54] Is a human life worth $10,000? Apparently the N.H.S. administrators feel that most lives are not. As Table 6-3 shows, human lives are considered far more valuable in most other industrialized nations.

Table 6-3

PATIENTS TREATED FOR CHRONIC RENAL FAILURE, DECEMBER 31, 1976

Country	New Patients Per million Population	Patients being treated by dialysis or with a functioning transplant Per Million Population
Austria	NA	65.8
Canada	NA	73.4[1]
Germany	30.8	105.0
France	30.3	111.3
Italy	27.6	102.0
Netherlands	21.4	108.5
Spain	14.4	39.3
Sweden	28.7	99.3
Switzerland	30.9	150.0
United Kingdom	15.1	71.2
United States	NA	120.0[2]

1. December 31, 1975.
2. Excludes transplants. The current U.S. figure, including transplants, is about 170 per million population.
Source: Office of Health Economics, *Renal Failure: A Priority in Health?* (London: Office of Health Economics, 1978), Table 7, p. 30. Data on Canada taken from Mary-Ann Rozbicki, *Rationing British Health Care: The Cost/Benefit Approach*, Executive Seminar in National and International Affairs, U.S. Department of State, April, 1978, p. 22. U.S. figure estimated from data provided by the Department of Health, Education and Welfare.

Scanners, dialysis machines and other complicated medical technology involve more than a capital expenditure. Equipment such as this also requires considerable current expenditure for technicians trained to use and operate it. It is for this reason that both of the above examples are probably more indicative of the second curious feature of British hospital care — the preference for routine and inexpensive treatment over modern medical technology.

Examples of the preference abound. The British press is filled with horror stories of children being denied critical care because of a lack of intensive care units in which to treat them.[55] In the Liverpool-Wellington area children in need of hole-in-the-heart surgery face a two-to-three-year wait — a wait which doctors believe may jeopardize their chance for survival. Many haemophilic children are denied treatment with Factor VIII, which prevents pain from haemorrhage into their joints.[56] And in some cases (such as spina bifida), children are simply allowed to die because the cost of continued treatment is considered to be too high.[57]

Pacemakers in Britain are in even shorter supply than dialysis machines.[58] Moreover, a great many people with life-threatening heart diseases are being turned away from hospitals or forced to wait for dangerously long periods of time. It is estimated that fifty people in Merseyside die each year while waiting for heart surgery, even though Mersey has one of the highest rates of heart surgery in Britain.[59] In the last decade, only ten heart transplants have been performed in all of Britain. By contrast, 150 transplants were performed at Stanford University Medical Center in California over the same period of time.[60]

On the whole, British hospital specialists have access to, and order, far fewer laboratory tests (such as X-rays, etc.) than do their U.S. counterparts. Much diagnostic and theraputic equipment is simply not available, and expenditures on high technology equipment are rigidly controlled. Many surgical specialities (and their associated physical plant) are found only in regional or teaching hospitals. Patients often have to travel a considerable distance for relatively unsophisticated treatment — provided they can travel and can gain admission.[61]

As an example of the limited supply of acute facilities, consider the conclusions of a recent survey of conditions in the field of cardiology:

> In the East Anglian Region, 1974 data show that, of the 2.67 acute beds available per 1,000 population, only 0.02 were earmarked for cardiology (the same as for dermatology and less than for plastic surgery). Moreover, the number was that high only because of the availability in Cambridge District hospitals; no beds were earmarked for cardiological patients in the entire Norfolk and Suffolk areas nor in the Peterborough District of Cambridgeshire. In the new hospital recently opened in York . . . there is a coronary care unit with a capability to computer-monitor eight or nine patients; the unit is served by general medical doctors "with an interest in cardiology", since not one staff member is a fully trained cardiological specialist.[62]

Heart disease, incidentally, is the second leading cause of days of incapacity and the leading cause of death in Britain.[63]

Another example of the limited supply of acute care facilities is in the area of emergency care. The old American advice, "never be sick on weekends or holidays," has double and quadruple force in Britain. One observer recently remarked that "if your dog is injured, there is a fifty percent chance that your vet has a radio-telephone link; but if *you* are injured, the odds are lowered to five percent."[64] Not only is the N.H.S. notoriously slow in responding to medical emergencies, but large areas (South East England, South Wales and Scotland) are largely without any immediate care facilities.[65]

It is necessary to emphasize that the limited supply of acute care facilities stems as much, or more, from conscious budget decisions as it does from the simple fact that the total N.H.S. budget is limited. For example, although the N.H.S. apparently spent only $40 million in 1976 treating patients with chronic renal failure, that same year it spent $48 million giving people "free" eyesight tests.[66] Similarly, although emergency care facilities are in short supply, only 1.5 million of the 21.7 million ambulance journeys provided in 1976 were for emergency purposes.[67] Since the overwhelming majority of ambulance rides had nothing to do with medical emergencies, it is not surprising that British ambulances rarely contain a paramedic or an emergency medical technician (EMT).[68] This situation contrasts dramatically with the U.S. experience, where ambulances are mainly used for medical emergencies and generally carry paramedics or EMTs.[69]

Another indication of British budget priorities is furnished by the new hospital in York. This hospital, as we noted above, has a limited coronary care unit and no fully-trained cardiological specialist. Yet the hospital features a complete gymnasium with a full-time therapist, a hydrotherapy unit with heated pool and mechanical lifting/dipping devices, a job-oriented industrial machine unit, handicrafts and other occupational therapy equipment, and a complete kitchen for self-help orientation.[70]

Clearly the British place far more emphasis on the "caring" and rehabilitative functions of their hospitals than on the "curing," and even life-saving, functions. They do so to a degree that would astonish and horrify most American observers. What is more, a movement is now underway to shift even more spending out of the "curing" and into the "caring" functions of the hospital sector.

The same Consultative Document which called on the N.H.S. to "put people before buildings" also called for a new shift in spending priorities. In the near future, the clear winners in the struggle for new hospital funds will be those who suffer from chronic illness (geriatrics, the mentally ill, and the handicapped.) The clear losers will be those who suffer acute illness.[71] We will examine some of the political motives behind these spending priorities in Chapter 10.

The Quality of Care: Hospital Incentives

As we saw in Chapter 4, deterioration in the quality of the good or service being produced almost always accompanies non-price rationing. Moreover, the greater the gap between the quantity demanded and the quantity supplied, the greater the deterioration in quality is likely to be. In Chapter 5, we saw considerable evidence of this proposition in the market for the services of general practitioners. The proposition is equally valid in the market for hospital services.

As former Minister of Health Enoch Powell has pointed out, deterioration in quality serves an important rationing function.[72]Along with the waiting list, a lower quality of service reduces the value of, and hence the demand for, medical care. Consequently, like the waiting list, a reduction in quality serves to solve the overall problem of excess demand.

Although quality deterioration mainly affects the demand for medical care, it comes about largely because of decisions on the supply side. Suppliers of medical care are prompted to reduce the quality of the services they offer for two reasons. First, by reducing the level of service offered to each patient treated, more patients may be provided with *some* treatment, given the available resources. In other words, lower quality allows a *larger volume* of patients — a result that is viewed as desirable by many in the medical community.

Second, the suppliers of medical care find that they suffer no penalty as a result of quality deterioration. Since there is ample excess demand for their services, they may reduce the quality of those services and still find the market ready to consume all that they have to offer. As a consequence, if the suppliers have any personal goals other than that of maintaining quality, it costs them nothing to pursue those goals. Since most of us have a great many personal goals other than maintaining the quality of our work, we should not be surprised to learn that members of the medical community are no different than we are in this respect.

In the British hospital sector, evidence of quality deterioration is pervasive. We shall organize our investigation of this phenomenon around the incentives faced by three distinct groups: (1) the N.H.S. and hospital administration; (2) hospital doctors; and (3) the hospital staff.

The fact that both hospital administrators and N.H.S. administrators are willing to sacrifice quality for volume is indicated by the general preference for current expenditure over capital expenditure. By eschewing the technology of modern medical science and opting for large increases in staff, N.H.S. hospitals have been able to handle larger and larger caseloads. This is one of the reasons why the number of patients treated each year more than doubled between 1949 and 1976, even though the number of hospital beds fell by 8 percent over the same time period.[73]

Another reason why the hospital caseload has increased is the lowering of the average length of time patients spend in hospitals. Average length of stay fell from 29 days in 1966 to 21.6 days in 1976.[74] In part, this is a commendable trend. Studies have shown that for many types of treatment, length of stay can be reduced without endangering the health of the patient. In Britain, however, with urgent cases on the waiting list, there have been "occasions when patients have [been] prematurely discharged in order to make room for others in more acute need."[75]

Perhaps a more important factor influencing the quality of care patients receive, however, is the fact that the interests of hospital personnel and the interests of patients often diverge. Some years ago, R. M. Titmus, an ardent supporter of socialized medicine, warned that "one of the new problems is the danger that the hospital may tend increasingly to be run in the interests of those working in and for the hospital rather than in the interests of the patients."[76]

A rather extreme confirmation of Titmus' fears was made public in 1977. Despite the widespread shortage of medical technology throughout the N.H.S., the British Veterinary Association admitted that year that between 200 and 250 cats and dogs were receiving cancer radiation treatment at N.H.S. hospitals, using the same facilities that were used for human patients. At least eight major hospitals were involved in what was cryptically described as an "unofficial" arrangement between vets and radiotherapists.[77]

Nor is this example an isolated one. Today there is ample evidence to confirm the early warning of Titmus. Michael Cooper has ably summarized what it all means for the patient:

Outpatient departments often seem to be run for the maximum convenience of consultants, whilst patients' time is valued at naught. Appointment systems which give everyone the same time still exist: the standard of comfort whilst waiting often compares unfavorably with British Rail waiting rooms. Inpatient conditions are much the same. Patients are too often treated as being uniformly stupid and afforded no privacy and little dignity. Once in bed the patient suffers an abnormal routine, with continuous anxiety-provoking activity all around him and only the barest minimum of information. These conditions can be tolerated for short spells (especially if the patient is too ill to care), but the long term patient for whom conditions are most important ironically suffers the worst physical facilities.

Few people when fit are prepared to stay in dormitory accommodations that are of such poor quality, with such a generally poor standard of food and general amenities. *In 1970, twenty-seven per cent of all known cases of food poisoning occurred in hospitals — more than in restaurants, clubs, and canteens put together.*[78]

The idea that hospitals are dangerous places in which to be was forcefully argued (and greatly exaggerated) in a recent book by Ivan Illich.[79] It is not surprising that one investigator would report that Illich "found a more sympathetic audience in Britain than in this country."[80] Well he might have. Not only do patients risk their health by consuming hospital food, they apparently also take great risks by consuming hospital-administered drugs. It is estimated that 30 percent of hospital patients suffer unwanted effects of hospital drugs.[81] For those who survive the hospital, it is not clear how beneficial the hospital treatment has been. An early study of N.H.S. hospitals concluded that two years after leaving the hospital, 36.3 percent of all patients are dead, and 56.6 percent of all patients are either dead or "unimproved".[82]

While there is little doubt that British hospitals have sacrificed quality for volume and for the interests of those who run the hospitals, quality of care is difficult to measure. An illustration of what may happen in the hospital on a day-to-day basis, however, was vividly recorded in a horrifying documentary shown on British television in May of 1978. The documentary consisted of film coverage of the activities on five consecutive days at King's College Hospital in London.

(Note: this distinguished teaching hospital is one of Britain's best, not one of its worst.) The following is a summary of the events recorded each day.[83]

Day 1:

A senior nurse admits to the film crew that patients have died due to insufficient nursing care, and that some patients would be safer if they stayed away from the hospital. "When the ambulance arrives," she adds, "they think they're saved. They don't realize their problems are only just beginning the minute they enter King's."

A patient, asked to come in for an operation, is kept waiting four hours before being sent home because no bed is available. A few hours later the patient is recalled. The senior nurse says this often happens.

The senior nurse in intensive care explains that there is normally only one nurse on duty at night who understands the complex machinery. Often she has to work with nurses who have never been in an intensive unit before, and who have no understanding of the procedures or of what to do in an emergency. She claims that some nurses are frightened of the equipment and accidentally misuse it.

Day 2:

In the orthopedic ward there are four nurses to care for 28 patients. The head nurse says the ward is literally unsafe.

Day 3:

A senior heart surgeon admits that errors by untrained nurses have caused the death of patients during emergencies.

A patient who has suffered several severe heart attacks is surrounded by expensive cardiac monitoring equipment. There are, however, no nurses available to check the readout and keep watch on his condition. A nurse admits that in an emergency the man could die without a nurse even being aware of it. In an attempt to deal with the lack of supervision, arrangements are made to transfer the man to the intensive care unit. He is kept waiting in a corridor outside the unit until it becomes clear that there will be no bed available that day. He is returned to his unsupervised room. A nurse tells him that plans have been changed because of his "improvement." She admits to the TV crew that she is getting used to lying to patients to avoid having them upset in such situations.

That evening the hospital is declared unsafe and closed to all new admissions — including emergencies.

Day 4:

The hospital reopens, but many due for admission that day are turned away for want of beds.

A head nurse explains that hospitals are now forced to use agency nurses to supplement their staff. The hospital telephones a central pool of nurses who work part-time and are sent to hospitals on a daily basis. The nurse claims that many of these nurses are very unreliable and, of course, do not know the patients. She also claims that many have daytime jobs and fall asleep on night duty.

Day 5:

There is a meeting of staff to protest the shortages.

A new patient is kept sitting in a waiting room for six hours for a bed to become vacant.

Senior doctors blame political decision to trim expenditures for the chaos at the hospital. One says of the situation at King's: "We don't actually have a notice on the door saying 'Take Care — This Place is Unsafe.' But I don't know why we don't!"

Some deficiencies in the quality of care administered in British hospitals are the result of a chaotic and inefficient system. Yet others are the result of conscious, premeditated decisions on the part of the N.H.S. administrators. The decision to skimp on modern medical technology is one example. The decision to allow the quality of hospital doctors and nurses to deteriorate is another.

The N.H.S. has caused the quality of its medical staff to deteriorate in two ways. First, the compensation for full-time hospital doctors is strikingly low by international standards. Second, it has sharply limited the number of consultant positions that it will fill. This is important, since hospital consultants receive the highest rates of pay and are the only hospital doctors permitted to engage in lucrative, part-time private practice. We shall look at these two decisions in more detail later. For the moment, our interest is in their consequences: many of the best and brightest hospital doctors are either fully or partially leaving the health service.

There has been a steady outflow of about 400 doctors each year to countries like the U.S., Australia, Canada and New Zealand.[84] This is equivalent to about 15 percent of the number graduated by British medical schools in 1974.[85] Of course the motive for emigration is not always financial. Many doctors coming to the U.S., for example, do so as much to escape the conditions of socialized medical practice as in search of higher income. Yet it is clear that government policy actually encourages the outflow.

Approximately 66 percent of all hospital consultants hold part-time appointments with the N.H.S.[86] The great bulk of these doctors engage in private practice, where the expected annual income can be substantial by British standards. The N.H.S. not only allows such practice, but actually encourages it by allowing private patients to be treated in government hospitals. This is a topic that will be examined extensively in Chapter 8.

As a consequence both of emigration and of private practice, there is a severe shortage (even by N.H.S. standards) of highly-trained doctors in N.H.S. hospitals. The shortage of surgeons is so bad in some areas of the country that those surgeons practicing there have been forced to limit their work to emergency and malignancy service only. Moreover, even in those areas of the country where the number of surgeons appears to be adequate, there is often a shortage of anaesthetists, radiologists and other specialist support staff.[87]

While Britain has been exporting about 400 of its own doctors each year, at the same time it imports an equal number of foreign doctors from countries like India and Nigeria. The irony in this is that, while British medical students may be well trained,[88] the imported doctors are on the whole very poorly trained. This fact only became public in 1975 when, for the first time, newly arrived doctors were given qualifying tests in medical knowledge and in the ability to communicate in English. Of those tested in the first six months, only about one-third passed.[89] By inference, the results suggested that about two-thirds of the foreign doctors practicing were unqualified to hold their hospital posts. What made these results so shocking was that 30 percent of all hospital doctors,[90] and 50 percent of all junior grade doctors at that time, were foreign-born.[91]

It might seem that the logical solution to the problem is to raise the incentives for British-trained doctors to practice in the N.H.S. But this is apparently not the solution the N.H.S. prefers. In fact, soon after the examinations were given, the *British Medical Journal* speculated that the standard of clinical knowledge required in the tests might have to be lowered in order to produce adequate numbers of foreign doctors for N.H.S. hospitals.[92]

Just as the N.H.S. policies have led to a deterioration in the quality of doctors, so have N.H.S. policies led to a deterioration in the quality of the hospital staff. In 1975, many hospitals reduced the years of training required for nurses from three to two years.[93] What is more, the annual amount spent training a nurse is about 10 percent of the annual amount spent on the education of a college student. Even so, only 50 percent of the nurses are rated as "qualified" nurses. Nursing is also another area in which the N.H.S. relies heavily on foreigners. Over 15 percent of all nurses and 26 percent of all new entrants into nursing schools are foreign-born.[94]

A major problem with nurses and other members of the technical staff is the high volume of turnover. Even at Guy's Hospital in London, the turnover in nurses is rapid. Radiographics leave Guy's on the average after only 18 months of employment, and physiotherapists leave after 30 months.[95]

In an attempt to deal with the shortage of qualified nurses and the high rate of turnover among them, many hospitals have turned to the practice of hiring temporary nurses. In response to the demand, a booming private "rent-a-nurse" business now exists and operates much like the deputy doctor agencies we looked at in Chapter 5. Moreover, as in the case of deputy doctors, the rising number of temporary nurses has intensified the concern over the quality of nurses employed by the N.H.S.

To test the charge that the "rent-a-nurse" agencies are lax on credentials, a reporter for *The* (London) *Times* falsely posed as a nurse and applied for a job as a "temp." Although the reporter's only real experience with hospital life was when she had her appendix out at the age of 14, she was promptly hired and told to report to the intensive care unit of a major hospital.[96] The same expose also discovered other abuses which should give potential patients cause for concern:

> We have discovered instances where temporary nurses have been unfamiliar with doctors' descriptions of variously named drugs; where they have been ignorant of new techniques because of gaps in their nursing career; and where they have shown a reluctance, because of the nature of their work, to familiarize themselves with a particular hospital's practices.[97]

To the degree that hospital administrators do bear a cost as a result of allowing quality deterioration, this cost is likely to be one which stems from patient complaints and, perhaps, public outrage. As a consequence, we would expect to find the quality of care the lowest in those sectors of the hospital service where patient complaints and public awareness of the problems are likely to be at a minimum. The evidence is consistent with this prediction — the worst care is administered to the elderly and the mentally handicapped.[98]

Certainly the evidence suggests that, on the average, the worst doctors gravitate to these fields. In 1975, 85 percent of the junior grade doctors in geriatrics and 86 percent in mental health were trained in foreign countries.[99] The evidence also suggests that the incentives for the best doctors to enter the field are weak. Geriatrics and mental health are two of the three specialties where consultants earned the smallest number of pay-enhancing awards.[100]

The conditions faced by patients in these fields, however, are far more serious than the quality of the doctors who attend them. As late as 1972, the Director of the Hospital Advisory Service was able to say that "it is possible to find wards in mental hospitals where patients sleep, eat, excrete, live and die in one large room."[101] A year later, a (London) *Times* exposé revealed that things had improved very little.[102]

In some mental wards, the annual cost of maintaining each patient is less than the annual cost of maintaining an inmate in British prisons. For the whole N.H.S., catering costs in 1973 averaged £3.58 per week per patient in mental wards, while the comparable sum for a patient in a London teaching hospital was £12.68. This is a difference that cannot be explained by variations in dietary needs.[103]

Some idea of the quality of treatment received is indicated by the following statistics: On the average, there is approximately one doctor for every 660 mentally ill patients in N.H.S. hospitals.[104] Moreover, mentally-ill patients, who fill 45 percent of all occupied beds, receive an average attendance of one hour per year per patient from hospital doctors. As one commentator observed, "it would be extraordinary indeed if patients did not suffer from delays in prescribing, in monitoring side effects, in over-treatment and in discharge following recovery" under these conditions.[105]

The Quality of Care: Doctor Incentives

One major difference between British medical students and American medical students is that in Britain, a specific term of training and the passing of examinations do not win for the student a qualification as a specialist. Full status as a specialist comes only with the appointment to a consultant position and, as we have seen, the number of such positions has been tightly limited in the N.H.S.

Following medical school, hospital doctors can expect to spend one year as a house officer and then progress to senior house officers. (House officers are equivalent to interns and junior residents in the United States.) The next two stages in the progression to consultant are registrar and senior registrar.

All junior doctors are theoretically undergoing training as specialists and, as such, they work under the supervision of a consultant. A cause of much bitterness in the hospital sector is the fact that junior doctors may work well into their middle 30's before they receive an appointment as a consultant. Moreover, even at that age many of them will be forced to abandon their specialty for general practice, or transfer to specialties where there are more openings for consultant positions.[106]

Once the coveted consultant status is achieved, the doctor will find that he occupies a position of considerable power within the hospital. He will also enjoy a large entourage of junior doctors, many of them highly trained, who do most of the work. In fact, so powerful is the position of consultant that the hospital service has been described as consisting of

> a series of personal empires of lordly consultants who are specialists in different fields, and who have lower-ranked doctors — many of them in their thirties and even some in their forties — serving under them. It is interesting that the consultant and his underlings are known as a "firm," and that the consultant is supreme in his medical empire, secure in his job for life, and accountable to almost no one.[107]

The major complaint of junior doctors is that they are overworked and underpaid. Table 6-4 reproduces some results of a study by Christopher Birt, a specialist in community medicine, of the workload for junior hospital doctors in the north of England during 1975. Within these broad results, there was considerable variation. In some cases, the workload was beyond any reasonable level. Surgical registrars in Trafford, for instance, averaged 125 hours per week. Birt summarized the conditions in the north of England in the following way:

> Junior hospital doctors were required to be on duty for rather more than twice what would normally be accepted as standard working hours, and they found themselves actually working at least 75% of this time.[108]

Table 6-4

WORKLOADS FOR JUNIOR HOSPITAL DOCTORS

Town	Hours of Duty/Week	Hours Actually Spent Working
Lancaster	93.4	66.3
Preston	87.9	68.5
Burnley	91.3	69.1
Manchester (central)	68.9	53.2
Rochdale	92.3	68.6
Stockport	85.0	70.3
Wigan	95.4	77.6
Trafford	96.3	69.2

Source: Taken from Stuart Butler, "Thirty Years of National Health Care: A Review of the British Experience," (Washington, D.C.: The Heritage Foundation, 1978), Table 3, p. 8.

In return for these hours, the junior doctors receive meager rates of pay. In 1978, for example, house officers were paid between $7,326 and $8,204. Registrars received between $8,204 and $10,218. And the salaries for senior registrars ranged from $9,636 to $12,558.[109]

If consultant status is achieved, the income-earning prospects for the junior doctor are somewhat better. Consultant's pay for full-time service ranges from $15,000 to $21,378. These salaries may be enhanced, however, by the receipt of merit awards. The awards are made by a select group of doctors, and are often based upon the opinions of the consultant's peers. These awards, which are known only to the individual consultant and his employer, may raise the consultant's annual pay to a maximum of $36,000. About three-fourths of the N.H.S. consultants earn the maximum base scale of $21,378, and one in three receives merit pay in some amount.[110]

As we noted above, consultant status also entitles the doctor to work part-time for the N.H.S. and engage in a private practice. About 25 percent of the consultants in 1978, for example, were working under "maximum part-time" arrangements. The consultant is paid nine-elevenths of a full salary, and is expected to be available to N.H.S. patients for 3½-hour sessions morning and afternoon, Monday through Friday, and in the morning on Saturday.[111]

There is no doubt that some British consultants do very well. For example, it appears that those with a very good private practice can earn between $50,000 and $70,000.[112] Only a small minority of doctors will earn incomes in this range, however. One way to appreciate the income picture facing most hospital doctors is to contrast physician incomes in Britain with those in the United States. In 1976, the median earnings of all hospital doctors in the U.S. was $62,800.[113] Since average wages in Britain are about one-half what they are in the U.S., for a British doctor to do as well by British standards he would have had to earn $31,400 that year. Yet to have achieved this salary, the full-time N.H.S. doctor would have had to be a consultant who had received the very highest merit award — an award given to only one percent of all consultants.[114] Of course, many of the best consultants will have a private practice. But it is estimated that the average part-time consultant earns only 18 percent more than the average full-time consultant.[115]

A more direct way of evaluating doctors' incomes in Britain is to compare them to the average wage paid in manufacturing. This is done in column three of Table 6-5 for the United Kingdom and for other countries as well. As the table shows, by this standard British doctors are the lowest paid among all industrialized countries!

British hospital doctors, then, work long hours, receive low average rates of pay and, as we have seen, frequently operate with a shortage of equipment and an inadequately trained and inadequately manned technical staff. The result has been a serious morale problem in N.H.S. hospitals. In fact, morale has been so low that British newspapers frequently and freely refer to the "breakdown" or the "collapse" of the N.H.S.[116]

How have these conditions affected the quality of work performed by British doctors? The judgment of Professor Harry Swartz on the quality of general practitioners probably applies with equal force to the hospital sector:

> It is a quality of medicine that varies from the excellent, personalized, compassionate and technically superb to uncaring travesties of health care, sometimes delivered by a foreigner whose English is none too good, and who dislikes his patients as much as they dislike him.[117]

One generalization, though, seems valid: in the hospital sector, as elsewhere in the N.H.S., doctors have little incentive to care about the attitudes, feelings and wishes of patients. Even if doctors care very much about the technical aspects of their work, they have little reason to care about the non-technical. For as Anthony Culyer has pointed out, "neither doctors' income nor their professional standing normally depends upon concern for the whole patient."[118] But this is an inherent

Table 6-5
DOCTORS' INCOME IN RELATION TO GROSS DOMESTIC PRODUCT (GDP) PER HEAD
(1974 or near date)

Country	GDP per head	Ratio of doctors' income to: Compensation of employees/ per employee	Average pro- duction worker gross earnings
Belgium			
Physicians and dentists	6.3	3.7	5.2
Pharmacists	6.0	3.6	4.9
Canada	6.8	5.0	4.8
Denmark (1973)	5.7	4.0	3.8
Finland (1970)	5.2	5.0	4.2
France	7.0	4.3	7.0
Germany (1973)	8.5	5.6	6.1
Ireland (1973)	7.6	3.7	3.5
Italy (1973)	9.5	4.3	6.8
Netherlands (1973)	10.2¹	5.0	6.3
New Zealand			
Physicians	6.2	4.0	3.9
Dentists	4.9	3.1	3.1
Norway	3.4	2.4	2.4
Sweden	4.6	3.3	3.5
United Kingdom (1973)	4.5	3.3	2.7
United States			
Physicians	6.7	4.5	5.6
Dentists (1972)	5.6	3.3	4.1

1. If GDP per person employed were used as the basis for this comparison, this apparent difference from other countries would be considerably reduced.

Source: Organization for Economic Cooperation and Development, *Public Expenditure on Health* (Paris: OECD, 1977), Table 9, p. 24.

feature of socialized medical care. Reflecting on his tenure as Minister of Health in the early 1960s, Enoch Powell explains why:

> I remember how strange it used to seem to me that ministerial circulars should be required in the 1960s to inculcate into hospital doctors and administrators — I suspect with little practical effect in the event — the desirability and methods of maintaining the most elementary and even courteous communications with the family doctors and their patients. *Alas, they do not need to do so.*[119]

What incentives do hospital doctors have to maintain the technical quality of their work? The incentives are mixed. On the one hand, doctors who achieve a high level of skill can look forward to pay-enhancing merit awards. On the other hand, as we shall see below, the doctor who allows his work to deteriorate has little to fear from malpractice suits, and probably even less to fear from reprisals by hospital administrators.

These mixed incentives appear to have produced mixed results. While Britain has some of the best doctors and best hospitals in the world, the performance of many doctors and hospitals falls well below the standards most Americans have come to expect. One area in which extensive monitoring of the quality of care administered has been carried out is that of maternity deaths. A 1972 government study concluded that 56 percent of the deaths in England and Wales had "avoidable factors."[120] In Scotland, one-third of the deaths were judged avoidable, and in half of these, doctors were found to be wholly or partly responsible.[121] Another study of coronary cases found that doctors arrive to administer treatment an average of four hours after the beginning of symptoms — by this time 50 percent of the patients are dead.[122]

The quality of patient care is now being increasingly threatened for another reason: slowdowns and strikes by hospital doctors. Although this is a tactic mainly adopted by non-medical staff workers, doctors have been using it too with increasing frequency. In 1975, for example, consultants staged a slowdown in a dispute with the government over the status of private beds in N.H.S. hospitals. That same year, in a dispute over pay and working conditions, junior doctors in many hospitals closed down the emergency rooms after 5 p.m. In many of these hospitals, however, the consultants, despite their own grievances, went on duty to make some emergency services possible.[123]

Aside from collective strikes and slowdowns, there is also the possibility of a unilateral strike. Dr. Derrick Henderson has described a rather extreme case, but one which vividly illustrates the incentives which British physicians face. This case involves a successful surgeon in a large city:

He went off in his Jaguar to do his twice monthly list in the provincial hospital nearby. He drove through rolling hills and glens, past the babbling brooks, and never arrived. The patients were premedicated and one was even anesthetized. The OR crew were standing by to swing into the fast action always demanded by the mercurial man.

He didn't show up. There were telephone calls — yes he *had* left for the hospital, no there were no reported automobile accidents. The crew stood down. The patients woke up. Have I had my operation? No, you haven't had your operation.

The police telephoned: they had located the surgeon. His car was parked down a dirt road beside a stream and he was fishing. He explained later: "The water looked so inviting and the salmon were jumping. I just thought, what the hell, I'd rather fish today than operate."[124]

The Quality of Care: Incentives of Hospital Workers

Morale problems for the thousands of workers in N.H.S. hospitals appear to be as severe as they are for the junior doctors. A great many complaints concern rates of pay. But the most demoralizing aspects of hospital work are not financial. Instead, they arise from the conditions of the work itself.

A recent report by the Royal College of Nurses gave vent to the frustration felt by nurses who are so understaffed that they cannot adequately do their jobs. The report attacked conditions in British hospitals and claimed that the health of patients is now at risk. The following replies to questionnaires sent out by the college show the despair prevalent among the hospital nurses:[125]

Nurse A:

Care has now become something that many people talk about but few are able to give in adequate amounts. Perhaps the government is waiting for a high level of statistics of patients who have come to harm in hospitals; or the patient population to stage some form of revolution in desperate appeal against the privations they suffer.

Nurse B:
   Morale is low because not only are we understaffed but, as the work is not up to the standard we would like to give, there is no job satisfaction either.

Nurse C:
   The situation of the wards is becoming impossible. The nursing staff are becoming exhausted, physically and mentally. I wonder how long I personally can stand the strain of a continual battle to try to complete work.

   Reports such as these help explain why the turnover rates among nurses and members of the technical staff are so high in British hospitals. Even the most conscientious among them soon realizes that there is little incentive, beyond personal satisfaction, to strive for a high quality of patient care. And it is perhaps for this reason that members of the hospital staff have become more and more concerned with *personal* goals rather than patient well-being. As *The Economist* recently pointed out, even the most dedicated of hospital workers often appear to be "more concerned with the health service as a provider of jobs than as a means of caring for patients."[126]

   This attitude figures most prominently in the growing militancy of Britain's hospital workers unions. Prior to 1970, there was no serious attempt to use industrial action to improve wages and working conditions among hospital workers. But over the last decade, work stoppages, slowdowns and general strikes have become routine phenomena in the hospital sector.[127]

   One of the most militant unions is the National Union of Public Employees (NUPE). NUPE represents hospital porters and other unskilled workers who, although they have no medical training, are nontheless vital for the orderly functioning of any hospital. The union aggressively pursues ideological as well as economic goals. For instance, during a campaign to phase-out pay beds in N.H.S. hospitals, the union refused to assist in operations on private patients unless they were emergencies. Thus, consultant surgeons were "faced with the ignominy of telephoning union officials to explain the details of each case and requesting permission to be allowed to carry on an operation."[128]

   The following examples of union activity during 1978 illustrate how widespread, and even dangerous, the situation has become:

February 1978
   Porters at the Dulwich Hospital, South London, refused to

allow operations to take place because they did not like one of the senior nurses. According to the porters, she gave orders without always saying "please" and "thank-you," and did not allow enough time for tea-breaks. One porter complained that he was "upset" because he was asked to move a trolley before he had finished a cup of coffee. Another took objection to a nurse criticizing him for regularly wheeling his bicycle through an anteroom next to the operating theatre.[129] The effect of the porters' action was the cancellation and postponement of several major operations. One man with stomach cancer had to be moved to another hospital. Another postponed operation involved a man with a gangrenous leg.[130]

March 1978

Telephone operators manning switchboards in the Midlands of England were instructed by their unions to monitor calls by doctors and other staff. If they were not, in the opinion of the operators, "genuine," they were to pull out the plug. Doctors in the 210 hospitals involved claimed that the action was causing serious problems, and that the operators had no qualifications to judge the importance of a call.[131]

May 1978

Rebel nurses and staff, members of the Confederation of Health Service Employees, decided to take over the running of the 900-bed Brookwood mental hospital in Surrey. According to the union's regional secretary:

"The management team had an agreement with the branch to consult before any rise in charges [for a staff child-care center]. They failed to do this ... We are now setting up a workers' council to take over the running of the hospital under the auspices of the Health authority."[132]

October 1978

A wave of industrial actions prompted the following editorial comment by *The Economist:*

Whether or not anybody has yet died as a direct result of the latest labor dispute to hit the health service, there is no doubt that people with suspicious lumps cannot have them diagnosed; children's eye operations are being postponed; hip operations for the relief of pain have had to be cancelled. People are dying faster, even if they are not already dead, and the extra suffering of many not dying is very real.[133]

So powerful have the hospital unions become that the doctors' newspaper, *On Call,* now claims that the unions "can dictate how a hospital is to be run."[134] Clearly, it is not to be run in order to maximize the well-being of patients.

What Can Patients Do?

The potential patient in an N.H.S hospital faces prospects that look quite bleak from an American perspective. Depending upon his condition, and the condition of other patients in his area, he faces a waiting list that may defer hospital admission for years. Once in the hospital, he faces a raft of contingencies that range from food poisoning and adverse drug reactions to the possibility that the entire hospital may be closed in a labor dispute. Given that he receives care, he runs the risks of doctor negligence and the consequences of being attended by an undertrained and understaffed corps of nurses and technicians. Under these circumstances, what alternatives are left open to the patient?

One solution to the waiting list problem was discovered in 1977 by a gallbladder patient named Rita Ward. Mrs. Ward, it seems, had been in great pain for 20 months. She had been on the hospital waiting list for 18 months, and had been told that a bed would not be available for at least another 12 months "because of the cutbacks."

Mrs. Ward had different ideas. Helped by her husband, her two daughters and three friends, she half-walked and was half-carried one morning into Britain's Northhampton General Hospital. The group found its way to the surgical ward where they happened to know that there was one empty bed available. Mrs. Ward promptly took off her clothes, climbed into bed, and announced she wasn't leaving until she had the operation which she had been told was necessary. "The only way to get me out of here," said Mrs. Ward from her hijacked bed, "is in a wooden box."

The case attracted nationwide publicity and created great consternation among hospital officials. After all, to have thrown her out on the street would have seemed inhumane. On the other hand, to have agreed to the operation might have "opened the floodgates." Eventually they operated.[135]

Clearly, the vast majority of patients on waiting lists cannot benefit from the "Ward Solution." Nonetheless, other options do exist. A certain percentage of beds called "pay beds" in N.H.S hospitals are reserved for the private treatment of patients. In addition, there are a number of private hospitals in Britain. Patients who choose the private option must not only pay their doctors for services rendered, but also pay the daily cost of their bed plus the cost of drugs they use. In Mrs. Ward's case, for example, the cost would have been about $80 per day.

The great benefit of the private option is that waiting times are greatly reduced, and sometimes nonexistent. Frequently, for example, patients can arrange for an operation on a specific day or week chosen for *their* convenience, rather than for the convenience of the N.H.S. The private option also solves the problem of the quality of care. The private patient knows precisely who will be operating and who will be assisting — these choices, after all, are his own rather than those of the N.H.S. bureaucracy. The option of private care, however, (which will be examined in Chapter 8) is an option open to only a small minority of the British population.

Another possible option is a blackmarket (or illegal) agreement. It is rumored that one way of moving to the head of a waiting list is by illegally compensating the doctor, who then *reconsiders* the urgency of the patient's condition. But, as in the case of the general practitioner, the opportunities here are not a matter of general public knowledge.

Beyond the patients' ability to secure better care by paying for it, the options open to patients are not promising. In theory, all hospitals have procedures whereby patients may complain about their treatment. These complaints are lodged with health authorities who have the power to discipline doctors if they find that such discipline is warranted.[136] A 1973 government report, however, discovered that only 43 percent of hospitals include information on the complaint procedure in their admissions book.[137]

A final option open to the patient is the civil suit. Under British law, malpractice is defined in much the same way as it is in the United States.[138] Moreover, since hospital doctors, unlike general practitioners, are employees of the N.H.S., the N.H.S. may be sued along with a doctor on the theory that the employer is vicariously liable for the actions of the employee.[139]

At this point, however, the similarities with American malpractice suits radically diverge. In Britain, jury trials in personal injury cases are very rare.[140] Furthermore, lawyers, whether barristers or solicitors, are not permitted to accept work on a contingency fee.[141] Add to this the fact that, since the N.H.S. is often a defendant in malpractice suits, the government has an interest in minimizing their impact. The upshot is that British malpractice awards are shockingly minor by U.S. standards.

In order to appreciate the contrast between the two systems, consider the case of *Williams v. City of Detroit,*[142] where an award of $750,000 was made for the death of a six-year-old boy following a delay in treating his fractured skull. In Britain, assuming a verdict of negligence is obtained (and it is by no means clear that it would be obtained!), the award would be about $1,500 plus funeral expenses! No attempt would be made to evaluate the parents' pain and suffering, and the damages in such a case would be intended as nothing more than a "token payment in respect of loss of expectation of life."[143]

Ironically, while the awards for the death of a child are meager, the awards given to those who live can be substantial. One British malpractice award was made for $170,000 in a case where the victim was forced to live with the injury. The general system of making awards has provoked one investigator to comment: "The U.K. attitude is open to criticism on the basis that, as regards children and adults without dependents, it is in general cheaper to kill than to maim."[144]

Who Receives Care?

During World War II, Prime Minister Winston Churchill had a glittering prize to offer his people for the postwar period:

Our policy is to create a national health service in order to secure that everybody in the country, irrespective of means, age, sex, or occupation, shall have equal opportunities to benefit from the best and most up-to-date medical and allied services available.[145]

To say that the N.H.S. has reneged on Churchill's promise is an understatement. At least in the hospital sector, inequality in the availability of medical resources is as great in Britain today as it was after the First World War.[146] Thirty years after the N.H.S. was founded, one commentator described the distribution of hospital services in the following way:

Anyone fortunate enough to live within the shadow of a great teaching hospital such as St Thomas's in London has the benefit of medical and surgical skills as good as any in the world. It is a different story in the industrial wastelands of the northwest of England, where waiting lists are long and many of the hospitals are worn out Victorian buildings, ill-equipped and understaffed.[147]

Figure 6-2 shows some of the gross inequalities that exist in the level of provision of hospital services across the hospital regions of England and Wales. This pattern has changed little since the N.H.S. was founded. As Ruth Levitt has observed, "those regions which were comparatively well provided at the start of the N.H.S. received allocations sufficient to preserve their advantages, so the less well-off ones could not make up the ground between them.[148]

Figure 6-2
REGIONAL VARIATIONS

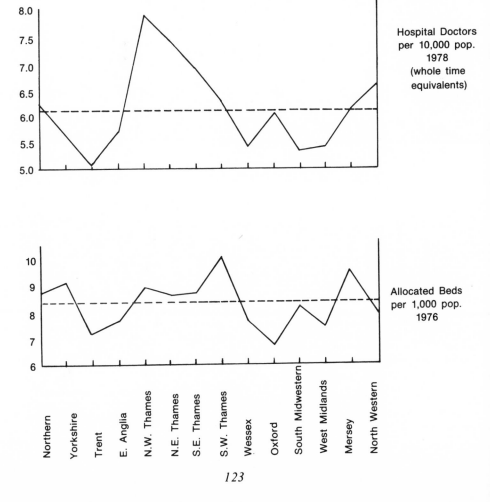

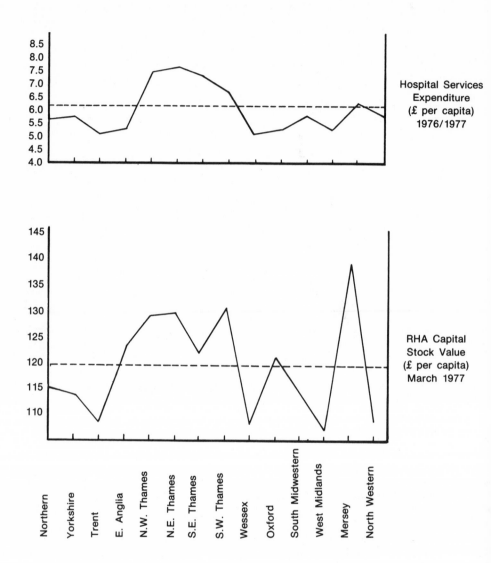

Source: For hospital doctors (whole time equivalents) per 10,000 population, and
   Hospital Services Expenditure (£ per capita) 1976/1977, data taken from
   Royal Commission on the National Health Service Report, (chairman: Sir
   Alec Merrison) (London: Her Majesty's Stationery Office, July, 1979), Table
   3.2, p. 16 and Table 3.1, p. 15.
   For allocated beds per 1,000 population, data taken from Department of
   Health and Social Security, *Health and Personal Social Services Statistics
   for England* 1977 (London: Her Majesty's Stationery Office, 1977), Table
   4.10, p. 83.

For RHA capital stock value (March 1977), data taken from Department of Health and Social Security, *Sharing Resources for Health in England: Report of the Resource Allocation Working Party* (London: Her Majesty's Stationery Office, 1976), Table D5, p. 128. Regional population statistics taken from Department of Health and Social Security, *Health and Personal Social Services Statistics* 1977, (London: Her Majesty's Stationery Office, 1977), Table 1.3, p. 15.

Regional variations in hospital waiting lists are depicted in Table 6-6. The pattern of inequalities here is much the same as that in Figure 6-2. As the table shows, the waiting list per capita varies over 100 percent from the lowest to the highest region.

Table 6-6

REGIONAL WAITING LISTS
(England and Wales, 1971)

Regional Hospital Board	list per 1,000 population	list per consultant	size of list
South Western	14.3	66.1	45,334
Manchester	14.2	74.7	65,101
N.W. Metropolitan	12.3	28.4	52,194
Birmingham	11.9	59.2	60,774
Oxford	11.8	51.0	23,602
Wales	11.8	60.2	32,161
Sheffield	10.5	64.8	48,725
S.E. Metropolitan	10.3	35.8	35,170
Newcastle	10.2	43.4	31,021
Liverpool	9.7	34.9	21,424
N.E. Metropolitan	9.5	33.7	30,911
Wessex	8.9	47.5	18,191
S.W. Metropolitan	8.5	26.6	28,668
East Anglia	8.5	38.5	15,058
Leeds	7.0	34.9	22,586

Source: A.J. Culyer and J.G. Cullis, *New Society*, 16 August, 1973. This first appeared in *New Society*, London, the weekly review of the Social Sciences.

In some ways, though, Figure 6-2 and Table 6-6 present a picture of much more equality than actually exists. This is because the variations *within* a region are often much greater than between regions.[149] For example, Figure 6-2 indicates that those regions which receive the most per capita hospital spending are about 24 percent above the national average, while those regions which receive the least per capita spending are about 24 percent below the national average. Actual variations between hospital districts are in fact much greater than this.

More detailed data relating to area health authorities have been analyzed by Buxton and Klein.[150] Their main results are summarized in Table 6-7. As the Table indicates, the total range of per capita spending varies from 62 percent above the national average in Liverpool to 69 percent below the average in Sandwell. Even greater variations evidently exist in individual specialties.

Another, more comprehensive study of inequalities in the provision of care was conducted by two British economists, Michael Cooper and Anthony Culyer.[151] This study focused on the fourteen health regions, and constructed 31 indices of hospital care, such as the number of consultants, the number of teaching hospitals, the number of a specific type of operation, etc.

One of the interesting findings of this study was that there are greater variations in manpower between regions than there are in per capita spending. For example, Cooper and Culyer found that the Newcastle Region had twice as many gynecologists per female as did the Sheffield Region; Birmingham had twice as many whole time equivalent consultants as Sheffield; and Liverpool had twice as many psychiatrists as Manchester. What is more, the study found no evidence of one variable compensating for another. Areas relatively deprived by one yardstick were regularly deprived by others. The economists found a high degree of correlation between doctors' salaries per patient per week and nurses' salaries; between doctors' salaries and expenditure on equipment; and between expenditure on equipment and expenditure on pharmaceuticals.

Also interesting is the distribution of teaching hospitals. These are the so-called *centers of excellence,* with high concentrations of consultants who hold the very highest merit awards. The Wessex Region had no such hospital, while the North Western Metropolitan Region had one teaching hospital bed for every 650 people.

Is it possible that those areas which are relatively well-endowed with hospital services are those areas which have the greatest medical need? In fact, the reverse is true. As in the case of the distribution of general practitioners, the distribution of hospital resources seems to obey the "inverse care" law. Insofar as *need* is indicated by crude morality and morbidity statistics, "current provision appears to bear an almost inverse relationship to need."[152]

This is a remarkable outcome in a system of health care that has been socialized for over 30 years. Why has it happened? The unequal distribution of hospital services is in part the result of political pressures faced by the government and the N.H.S. administrators. These are pressures that we will examine in Chapter 10. The unequal dis-

Table 6-7

VARIATIONS IN HOSPITAL SPENDING BY AREA HEALTH AUTHORITIES, 1971-72

	Pop. (1000s)	Current expenditure	Total	General medicine	General surgery	Traumatic and ortho-paedic surgery	Mental handicap	Mental illness	Maternity	Maternity (adjusted)†	Geriatric and chronic sick	Geriatric and chronic sick (adjusted)‡
						%Variation from National Average for Provision *per Capita* — BEDS						
Mersey												
Cheshire	865	-11	39	-25	0	28	77	122	-17	-18	42	65
Liverpool*	607	62	38	192	130	90	-47	-69	99	105	31	36
St. Helens and Knowsley	377	-34	13	5	-25	-12	-100	165	-43	-44	-60	-55
Sefton	425	-15	-6	71	23	-1	19	-90	-12	-10	-18	-19
Wirral	355	-10	-2	60	85	95	-86	-77	17	21	-23	-40
Oxford												
Berkshire	624	-10	1	-11	1	7	49	-37	27	20	-19	1
Buckinghamshire	477	-29	-24	-29	-33	-54	-54	-39	9	5	-23	-9
Northamptonshire	468	-32	-15	-36	-9	17	-59	-24	-9	-8	49	53
Oxfordshire*	505	3	24	-21	-19	60	71	43	6	2	-19	-5
South Western												
Avon*	901	14	23	33	-7	32	190	-42	36	37	-5	-9
Cornwall	378	-30	-7	-38	-41	-30	-39	31	-5	4	24	-6
Devon	896	-14	14	-32	0	-18	46	18	6	18	24	-11
Gloucestershire	467	-36	-18	-45	-22	5	-100	4	18	21	10	9
Somerset	386	-17	21	-44	-38	-40	29	77	17	26	66	40
S.W. Thames												
Croydon	334	N.A.	35	N.A.	N.A.	N.A.	331	4	0	N.A.	0	5
Kingston and Richmond	250	N.A.	30	N.A.	N.A.	N.A.	-13	170	-9	N.A.	-38	-44
Merton, Sutton and Wandsworth*	680	N.A.	58	N.A.	N.A.	N.A.	40	105	26	N.A.	29	17
Surrey	1111	N.A.	32	N.A.	N.A.	N.A.	124	86	4	N.A.	-23	-20
West Sussex	627	N.A.	-19	N.A.	N.A.	N.A.	-28	11	1	N.A.	-34	-56
Trent												
Barnsley	225	-51	-55	-22	-29	-31	-100	-88	-8	-7	-29	-20
Derbyshire	885	-37	-31	-63	-45	-39	-45	-21	-29	-28	-12	-9
Doncaster	280	-18	-15	-29	-7	-14	69	-64	56	54	-12	7
Leicestershire*	798	-40	-27	-63	-31	-58	-13	-26	-9	-10	-15	-8
Lincolnshire	503	-14	16	-36	-6	-8	58	35	2	5	-1	-5
Nottinghamshire*	973	-17	-23	-28	-10	4	-53	-31	-21	-21	-15	-5
Rotherham	243	-62	-60	-57	-39	-65	-100	-100	-33	-34	-5	16
Sheffield*	572	34	20	12	22	43	19	-2	32	38	34	32
Wessex												
Dorset	554	-18	10	N.A.	N.A.	N.A.	-39	63	-5	8	36	-12
Hampshire*	1353	-21	-4	N.A.	N.A.	N.A.	-13	46	-15	-17	-25	-22
Isle of Wight	110	-12	6	N.A.	N.A.	N.A.	-14	52	-41	-28	19	-24
Wiltshire	676	-10	5	N.A.	N.A.	N.A.	-26	4	9	10	56	53
West Midlands												
Birmingham*	1098	10	4	2	8	34	-28	0	14	20	20	25
Coventry	337	-30	-44	-24	-24	21	-100	-95	8	7	-25	-3
Dudley	294	-40	-40	18	22	-9	-56	-86	-18	-22	-33	-19
Hereford and Worcester	559	-12	46	-28	-13	-20	68	61	-7	-8	16	20
Sandwell	330	-69	-74	-57	-51	-60	-100	-100	-49	-47	-55	-49
Shropshire	337	-22	-3	-43	9	155	-95	-3	-1	-1	51	54
Solihull	192	20	74	-2	22	-38	292	21	114	96	-30	8
Staffordshire	962	N.A.	3	-35	-28	-5	-33	51	-17	-21	31	61
Walsall	273	-50	-10	-45	-8	-63	296	-100	-28	-31	-41	-17
Warwickshire	456	N.A.	9	-10	-6	-18	133	-8	-6	-11	23	54
Wolverhampton	268	N.A.	-37	-38	-12	-50	-100	-78	25	N.A.	-32	N.A.
Yorkshire												
Bradford	461	-13	10	18	3	-22	-11	-31	48	54	23	21
Calderdale	195	-33	-21	-5	-5	-12	-10	88	31	41	59	44
Humberside	838	-25	-7	-39	-15	-14	-12	-26	4	6	11	17
Kirklees	369	-13	15	N.A.	N.A.	N.A.	-86	95	56	63	55	51
Leeds*	737	2	0	4	-16	20	-15	-8	-15	-18	0	-1
N. Yorkshire	628	-15	21	-6	3	22	3	10	8	11	66	55
Wakefield	302	1	49	21	31	96	27	109	-3	11	38	51

*Teaching Area.
†Beds per female in age group 15-44.
‡Beds per person in age group 65 and over.
N.A.=Not available from profile.

Source: Buxton & Klein, "Distribution of Hospital Provision: Policy Themes and Resource Variations," *British Medical Journal*, February 8, 1975.

tribution of resources, however, is also the result of the way in which doctors and nurses have responded to N.H.S. policy.

As in the case of general practitioners (at least until recently), hospital doctors and nurses receive uniform rates of pay — regardless of where they choose to locate. This means that:

> the doctor who works in a surgical specialty in a pleasant south coast resort gets the same salary as his opposite number in a crowded, under-doctored city in the industrial north. The visiting district nurse in the Scottish Highlands gets the same salary as her counterpart in an overcrowded Midland city.[153]

Moreover, the very best doctors have added incentives to practice in areas that are already well-endowed with talent and medical services. For example, a disproportionate number of merit awards is held by doctors in teaching hospitals, whose geographical distribution is hardly egalitarian.[154] In addition, the right to treat private patients (who inevitably come from high-income groups) also induces doctors to locate where the need for their service is comparatively low.[155]

Economic Efficiency in the Hospital Sector

How does the hospital sector of the N.H.S. rank in terms of the standard of *economic efficiency?* Very poorly. One recent study found that the allocation of hospital beds among consultants was seriously out of line with their respective requirements and with their operating time. Another study found that patients were admitted on set days, irrespective of the amount of preparation needed, thus wasting the patients' time. Even in nonmedical areas, inefficiency abounds. For example, about one-fourth of the hospital budget goes for supplies and equipment. Yet suppliers complain of irregular and unplanned purchases, of duplicated orders, and of no coordination between departments within the same management area.[156]

But if management problems exist in the N.H.S. hospitals, they certainly do not stem from a lack of managers or clerical staff. As Table 6-8 shows, the size of the administrative and technical staffs in N.H.S. hospitals is skyrocketing. Over the decade from 1965 to 1975, the N.H.S. bureaucracy increased by 134 percent. Over the same period, the number of hospital doctors increased by only 29 percent.

Is it possible that all of these additional administrators and clerks add to the productivity of the hospital doctors, or perhaps to the productivity of the hospital as a whole? A recent study by two British health economists says *no.*[157] Anthony Culyer has made some cal-

Table 6-8

THE GROWTH OF N.H.S. BUREAUCRACY 1965-1976[1]

Year	No. of Doctors	No. of Administrators and Clerical Staff	Bureaucrat/Doctor Ratio
1965	39,497	42,164	1.07
1966	39,974	44,299	1.11
1967	40,895	45,667	1.12
1968	41,915	46,943	1.12
1969	42,857	49,193	1.15
1970	43,658	51,683	1.18
1971	45,192	54,509	1.21
1972	46,868	58,547	1.25
1973	48,200	62,620	1.30
1974	49,341	81,696	1.66
1975	50,993	97,596	1.91
1976	52,006	104,388	2.01

1. Figures are for England and Wales in each case. Part-time staff have been represented as full-time equivalents.
Source: Central Statistical Office, *Annual Abstract of Statistics*, 1973 and 1977 (London: Her Majesty's Stationery Office).

culations based on this study, and the results are summarized in Table 6-9.[158] Note that, by every measure of productivity chosen, the growth of productivity was negative over the period studied.

One statistic that health economists are paying more and more attention to in evaluating hospital efficiency is the length of time the average patient spends in the hospital once he is admitted. In general, the more inefficient the hospital, the longer the average length of stay will be. Health economist Victor Fuchs explains why:

> An important determinant [of length of stay] is the efficiency with which the staff carries out the necessary diagnostic and therapeutic procedures. Are there delays in conducting tests and taking X-rays? Do these have to be repeated because of errors? Are operating rooms available when needed? Do patients linger longer than necessary simply because their physicians are away or have forgotten to discharge them? Adverse side effects of drugs, tests, and surgery also frequently increase the length of stay. One study of hospitalization for neurosurgery found that postoperative infection, which occured in 17 percent of the cases, extended the average stay an additional eighteen days.[159]

Of course, length-of-stay statistics are not foolproof indicators of efficiency. One way to reduce the average length of stay is to dis-

Table 6-9

HOSPITAL AVERAGE PRODUCTIVITY

(1960 = 100)

	1961	1962	1963	1964	1965	1966	1967	1968	1969	1970
Crude productivity Index (1) (deaths and discharges)	100.5	101.4	103.9	104.6	102.9	101.2	100.1	99.7	98.8	96.4
crude productivity Index (2) (with out-patient attendances)	101.1	99.7	102.3	103.6	101.0	99.7	98.9	97.8	97.5	95.7
social productivity	101.6	102.7	105.7	107.1	105.5	104.7	103.6	103.0	103.2	101.5
Economic output index (i) at 5% discount rate				100	97.3	92.3	92.9	91.3	93.0	87.9
(ii) at 10% discount rate				100	97.3	92.3	92.8	91.3	92.7	87.6
(iii) at 15% discount rate				100	97.2	92.2	92.8	91.3	92.6	87.5

Source: Anthony Culyer, *Need and the National Health Service* (Totowa, New Jersey: Rowman and Littlefield, 1976), Table 6.5, p. 75.

charge patients prematurely, thus endangering their health. We have seen that there are instances where N.H.S. hospitals, under the pressure of huge waiting lists, have done just that. In addition, "optimal" length of stay may vary radically from patient to patient because of important differences in their medical conditions. Nonetheless, numerous studies have confirmed that, on the average, patients spend way too much time in British hospitals. Studies conducted both in the United States and in Britain suggest that the average length of stay for a great many surgical procedures can be substantially shortened with no discernible health effects.[160] In fact, one specialist maintains that early discharge after surgery is actually better for the patients' health.[161]

Since the beginning of the N.H.S., average length of hospital stay has steadily declined. It fell from 49 days in 1949 to 34 days in 1961;[162] and, as Table 6-10 shows, the average stay in all hospitals had been reduced to 22.7 days in 1974. Nonetheless, length of stay in Britain is still *twice as high* as it is in the U.S. This difference between the two countries even extends to specific procedures like appendectomy and maternity cases, where the differences in the needs of patients are likely to be small. Average length of stay for patients with appendicitis is 10.3 days in Britain, while it is only 6.4 days in the U.S.[163] As Table 6-10 shows, length of stay for maternity cases is 64 percent higher in N.H.S. hospitals than in U.S. hospitals. This despite the paradoxical fact that Britain has more extensive home care services than exist in the U.S.[164]

One of the potentially misleading consequences of a lower average length of stay — and one of the reasons why many hospital administrators have weak incentives to try to achieve one — is that a lower average length of stay tends to raise the average cost per patient per day. One of the reasons why is illustrated in Figure 6-3. Patients who remain in the hospital long after an operation is performed are typically incurring only the "hotel" costs of the hospital — room and board. As the treatment costs are spread out over more and more days of mere recuperation, average cost per day becomes lower. On the other hand, early hospital discharge causes the treatment costs to be spread over only a few days of hospital stay. A second reason for this phenomenon is that short stays make life more difficult for hospital administrators and their staffs. It is usually difficult to keep occupancy rates up in the face of a rapid turnover of patients. Low occupancy rates, of course, mean that the fixed costs of the hospital will be spread over fewer patients per time period.[165]

Table 6-10
ADMISSION AND LENGTH OF IN-PATIENT SPELLS
(1974 or near date).

Country	Admission rate into hospitals (% of population)			Average stay in hospital (days)				
	All hospitals	General hospitals	Mental institutions	All hospitals	General hospitals	Mental institutions	Tuberculosis hospitals	Maternity hospitals
Austria	17.1	—	—	20.8	10.0	—	—	—
Belgium (1970)	10.7	9.9	.47	24.6	14.2	—	—	—
Canada (1973)	17.2	16.7	.27	18.8	10.0	419	100	5.6
Denmark (1970)	15.6	14.5	.64	18.8	12.8	119	30	—
Finland	18.2	13.8	.96	19.9	11.4	191	27	7.3
France (1973)	15.3	7.9	1.29	20.4	14.8	—	96	—
Germany	15.9	12.5	.31	20.2	17.1	198	85	9.8
Greece	10.7	7.2	.22	22.7	10.7	146	60	6.5
Ireland	—	9.9	—	14.5	11.0	—	68	—
Italy (1972)	16.2	—	—	—	—	—	—	—
Netherlands (1973)	10.7	10.0	.13	18.8	16.0	541	—	13.0
New Zealand (1970)	—	10.1	—	31.4	15.0	—	108	—
Norway	14.4	12.9	.24	29.0	11.4	339	67	8.3
Spain (1973)	7.3	6.6	.16	18.2	11.3	259	148	6.5
Sweden (1973)	17.9	15.8	.92	26.2	13.0	148	61	—
Switzerland[1]	13.1	11.9	.71	24.7	14.0	—	78	10.1
U.K. (England and Wales)	11.1	9.0	.32	22.7	12.6	319	23	6.9
United States	17.0	16.4	.30	11.1	8.3	143	89	4.2

Source: Organization for Economic Cooperation and Development, *Public Expenditure on Health Care* (Paris: OECD, 1977), Table 5, p. 19.

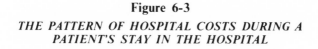

Figure 6-3

*THE PATTERN OF HOSPITAL COSTS DURING A
PATIENT'S STAY IN THE HOSPITAL*

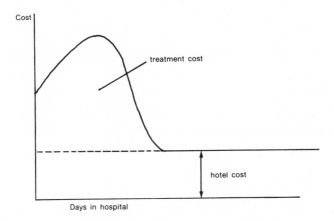

Source: C. J. Roberts, "Implications of Shortening the Time Spent in Hospital" in
Health Care in a Changing Setting: the U.K. Experience, CIBA Foundation
Symposium, No. 43 (Amsterdam: Elsevier, 1976), p. 56.

Other things being equal, then, an efficient hospital will tend to
have a high average cost per patient per day. Thus, it is ironic that
U.S. hospitals are routinely criticized for their high per patient per
day costs by those who advocate greater government regulation and
control of the hospital sector. What the critics overlook is that the
U.S. handles one of the highest admission rates in the world (see Table 6-10, Column 1), with fewer hospitals and fewer hospital beds per
capita than any other country (see Table 6-11). Were the N.H.S.
hospitals as efficient as U.S. hospitals, the British could reduce their
hospital capacity by over fifty percent and *still* handle the same
number of patients annually!

Corroborating evidence that British patients tend to stay in the
hospital too long was produced by a study that actually examined the
patients in the medical wards of a hospital in Birmingham. The study
concluded that 25 percent of the male patients and 42 percent of the
female patients had no therapeutic or diagnostic need to be there.
Even more alarming are studies which show that a large number of
patients in N.H.S. hospitals should never have been admitted in the
first place. One study found that as many as 40 percent of all acute

Table 6-11

PHYSICIANS AND BEDS, AN INTERNATIONAL COMPARISON

Country	MDs /10,000 pop.	Beds /10,000 pop.	Beds/MD
Australia	12.7	121.4	9.59
Belgium	15.9	83.0	5.19
Canada	15.0	98.1	6.55
Denmark	14.4	96.8	6.72
Finland	10.9	128.9	11.81
France	13.9	103.9	7.50
Germany, Federal Republic	17.8	112.6	6.31
Japan	11.6	127.8	11.04
Netherlands	13.2	70.7	5.37
Norway	14.5	130.8	8.99
Sweden	13.9	149.4	10.76
United Kingdom	13.6	109.1	7.30
United States	16.1	75.1	4.88

Source: Joseph P. Newhouse and George A. Goldberg, *Allocation of Resources in Medical Care from an Economic Viewpoint: Remarks to the XXIX World Assembly of the World Medical Association and Commentary* (Santa Monica, California: The Rand Corporation, 1976).

patients need not have been admitted on medical grounds.[166] This is an astounding finding in view of the fact that over half a million people were on hospital waiting lists at the time.

Not only is the average length of stay inordinately high in N.H.S. hospitals, but there is considerable, and almost inexplicable, variation in lengths of stay within the hospital sector. Average length of stay varies widely among the 14 health regions. But the variations are even larger among hospitals and among consultants. Comparisons of hospitals, for example, show that:

the variations between length of stay following treatment of hernia is fivefold, for appendicitis is sixfold, and for bronchitis and pneumonia ninefold. [One study] found that the removal of adenoids and tonsils from children over fifteen years old resulted in a six day stay for over eighty percent of all cases in one hospital group, but a stay of only one day in over fifty percent of the cases of another. [Another study] found that median duration of stay between consultants treating at least twenty peptic ulcers during one year ranged from six to twenty-six days, whilst that between physicians treating myocardial infarction from ten to thirty-six days.[167]

Another important source of inefficiency in the production of medical services is the process by which the type of treatment for specific medical conditions is chosen. Studies which show that injection therapy is a more economically efficient way of treating varicose veins than surgery, and those which show that kidney transplants are a "better buy" than dialysis, seem to have had little impact upon the decision makers.[168] Similarly, the decision to aim at having as many births as possible take place in hospitals seems to have been little influenced by cost-benefit analysis.[169] Recent financial cutbacks have slowed the development of health centers outside the hospital despite the fact that health centers have been shown capable of doing much of the work of hospital emergency rooms.[170]

Inefficiency also abounds in the way in which medical services are delivered to patients. It is by no means clear that the time and convenience of the hospital staff are more socially valuable than the time and convenience of patients. Yet we have seen that the former is routinely given priority over the latter in the hospital sector. As an additional example, take the case of renal dialysis. If the treatment were available in the evening, it would allow patients to continue uninterrupted with their daytime jobs. Yet in response to the demands of the hospital staff, this service is offered only during working hours.[171]

Not even the most ardent defender of socialized medicine would claim that N.H.S. dollars are spent in a way to maximize their social value. The lack of any coordinated "national clearing house" for waiting patients means that urgent patients wait in some areas, while elective surgery is performed in others. Thus, children wait a dangerous two or three years for hole-in-the-heart operations in Liverpool, while vacancies exist in other regions.[172] Surely economic efficiency as well as the nation's health could be improved if some of the 20.1 million non-emergency ambulance rides were sacrificed in favor of some additional dialysis machines or CAT scanners. Yet in the British health care system, this is not done.

Why is the hospital sector so inefficient? Part of the reason has to do with incentives. Neither hospital administrators nor doctors nor hospital staff, nor even patients, have an incentive, as individuals, to make things more efficient. Each of us acts on the basis of personal costs and personal benefits. Those who run the N.H.S. hospitals suffer no *personal cost* as a result of the abuses described above. Any major policy changes would undoubtedly make life less comfortable for them. Thus, as Professor Rudolf Klein has observed, cost-benefit analysis and other policy studies are resisted mightily by the N.H.S. bureaucracy.[173] Policy changes which would make the system more efficient are greeted with the same degree of enthusiasm as they are greeted by postal workers and teachers in the United States. Nor is there much political pressure to improve the efficiency of the hospital sector. We will see why this is so in Chapter 10.

Footnotes

1. Michael H. Cooper, *Rationing Health Care* (New York: Halsted Press, 1975), p. 99.
2. Economic Models, Ltd., *The British Health Care System* (Chicago: American Medical Association, 1976), p. 40.
3. Cooper, *Rationing Health Care*, p. 8.
4. Mary-Ann Rozbicki, *Rationing British Health Care: The Cost/Benefit Approach*, Executive Seminar in National and International Affairs, U.S. Department of State, April, 1978, p. 8.
5. Anthony J. Culyer, *Need and the National Health Service* (Totowa, New Jersey: Rowman and Littlefield, 1976), p. 100.
6. Interview with Lewellyn Rockwell, former editor of *Private Practice*, in *World Research INK*, March, 1979, p. 5.
7. *Royal Commission on the National Health Service Report* (Merrison Report) (London: Her Majesty's Stationery Office, 1979), p. 126.
8. Reported in the *Sunday Telegraph*, March 5, 1979.
9. Quoted in Anthony Lejeune, "Political Humbug," *Private Practice*, November, 1978, p. 78.
10. Culyer, *Need and the National Health Service*, p. 99.
11. *The* (London) *Times*, June 19, 1975, p. 4. Cited in Harry Swartz, "The Infirmity of British Medicine," in R. Emmett Tyrrell, Jr., ed., *The Future that Doesn't Work: Social Democracy's Failures in Britain* (New York: Doubleday, 1977), p. 29.
12. *British Medical Journal*, March, 22, 1975, p. 678.
13. *Ibid.*
14. Enoch Powell, *Medicine and Politics: 1975 and After* (New York: Pitman, 1976), p. 41.
15. Quoted in Lejeune, "Political Humbug," pp. 77-78.
16. The first survey of waiting patients was released in 1978. See *Royal Commission on the National Health Service: Patients' Attitudes to the Hospital Service*, Research Paper Number 5 (London: Her Majesty's Stationery Office, 1978).
17. Powell, *Medicine and Politics*, p. 40.
18. Cooper, *Rationing Health Care*, p. 22.
19. *Ibid*, p. 24.
20. For a personal account of such practices, see S.C. Hayward, *Managing the Health Service* (London: Allen and Unwin, 1974).
21. Powell, *Medicine and Policics*, p. 38.
22. *Ibid*, p. 39.
23. Martin S. Feldstein, *Economic Analysis for Health Service Efficiency* (Amsterdam: North-Holland, 1967).
24. A.J. Culyer and J.G. Cullis, "Hospital Waiting Lists and the Supply and Demand of Inpatient Care," *Social and Economic Administration*, vol. 9, 1975; and A.J. Culyer and J.G. Cullis, "Some Economics of Hospital Waiting Lists in the NHS," *Journal of Social Policy*, Vol. 4, 1976.
25. Powell, *Medicine and Politics*, p. 43.
26. *Ibid*, p. 39.
27. *Ibid.*
28. See the results of studies summarized in Cooper, *Rationing Health Care*, p. 54.
29. G. Forsyth and R.F.L. Logan, *Demand for Health Care* (Oxford: Nuffield Provincial Hospitals Trust, 1960).
30. Cooper, *Rationing Health Care*, p. 66.
31. Institute of Hospital Administrators, *Hospital Waiting Lists* (London, 1963.)
32. "An Affair of the Heart," *The Economist*, August 12, 1978, p. 17.
33. Swartz, "The Infirmity of British Medicine," p. 28.
34. Cooper, *Rationing Health Care*, p. 40.
35. *Ibid*, pp. 40-41.

36. Department of Health and Social Security, *Priorities for Health and Personal Social Services in England — A Consultative Document* (London: Her Majesty's Stationery Office, 1976).
37. Rozbicki, *Rationing British Health Care*, p. 15.
38. Stuart M. Butler and Eamonn F. Butler, *The British National Health Service in Theory and Practice: A Critical Analysis of Socialized Medicine* (Washington, D.C.: The Heritage Foundation, 1974), p. 30.
39. Cooper, *Rationing Health Care*, p. 36.
40. Stuart Butler, "Thirty Years of National Health Care: A Review of the British Experience" (Washington, D.C.: The Heritage Foundation, 1978), p. 15.
41. *Ibid.*
42. *Ibid.*
43. Economic Models, Ltd., *The British Health Care System*, p. 78.
44. Cooper, *Rationing Health Care*, p. 36.
45. D. Owen, *In Sickness and in Health: The Politics of Medicine* (London: Quartet Books, 1976), p. 32.
46. Cooper, *Rationing Health Care*, p. 33.
47. Joseph P. Newhouse and George A. Goldberg, *Allocation of Resources in Medical Care from an Economic Viewpoint: Remarks to the XXIX World Assembly of the World Medical Association and Commentary* (Santa Monica, California: The Rand Corporation, 1976), Table 4, p. 21.
48. *Ibid*, Table 5, p. 22.
49. Organization For Economic Cooperation and Development, *Public Expenditure on Health* (Paris: OECD,1977), pp. 25-26.
50. Swartz, "The Infirmity of British Medicine," p. 29.
51. Rozbicki, *Rationing British Health Care*, p. 9.
52. Data obtained from EMI, Ltd., London.
53. Rozbicki, *Rationing British Health Care*, pp. 10 and 22.
54. *Ibid.*
55. Dr. Tony Smith, "Verdict on the N.H.S.: Could do Better," *The* (London) *Times*, July 5, 1978.
56. Cooper, *Rationing Health Care*, pp. 92-93.
57. Rudolph Klein, "British Doctors Must Decide Whom to Save," *Chicago Tribune*, September 6, 1978.
58. Rozbicki, *Rationing British Health Care*, p. 9.
59. "Heart Surgery," *The Economist*, September 8, 1978.
60. "New Hearts for Old," *The Economist*, January 20, 1979.
61. Rozbicki, *Rationing British Health Care*, p. 9.
62. *Ibid.*
63. *Health and Personal Social Services Statistics*, pp. 172 and 16.
64. Cooper, *Rationing Health Care*, p. 112.
65. *Ibid*, pp. 102-103.
66. In 1976, the N.H.S. spent £24 million on eyesight tests. See Office of Health Economics, *OHE Briefing*, No. 7 (London: Office of Health Economics, 1978).
67. Department of Health & Social Security, *Health and Personal Social Services Statistics for England, 1977* (London: Her Majesty's Stationery Office, 1977) p. 127.
68. Arthur Gunawardena and Kenneth Lee, "Access and Efficiency in Medical Care: A Consideration of Accident and Emergency Services," in Keith Barnard & Kenneth Lee, eds., *Conflicts in the National Health Service* (London: Croom Helm, 1977), p. 218.
69. Every ambulance in the city of Baltimore, for example, carries a paramedic. Paramedics generally have more training than emergency medical technicians.
70. Rozbicki, *Rationing British Health Care*, p. 12.

71. Kenneth Lee, "Public Expenditure, Planning and Local Democracy," in Barnard and Lee, *Conflicts in the National Health Service*, p. 218.
72. Powell, *Medicine and Politics*, pp. 41-42.
73. Annabel Ferriman, "N.H.S. in Crisis 1: Doctors Complain of Chronic Under-Financing," *The* (London) *Times*, August 9, 1978.
74. *Ibid.*
75. "Diagnosis for A Cure: An Injection of Political Will," *The* (London) *Times*, May 20, 1973.
76. R.M. Titmus, *Essays on the Welfare State* (London: Allen and Unwin, 1963), p. 122.
77. Reported in Butler, "Thirty Years of National Health Care," p. 17.
78. Cooper, *Rationing Health Care,* pp. 93-94. (Emphasis added.)
79. Ivan Illich, *Medical Nemesis: The Expropriation of Health* (London: Marion Boyars, 1976).
80. Rozbicki, *Rationing Health Care*, p. 18.
81. Dr. Donald Gould, "Delivering Health Care Wisely and Well," *New Scientist*, April 7, 1977, p. 16.
82. Cooper, *Rationing Health Care,* p. 96.
83. *World in Action* (Independent Television) screened May 22, 1978. Reported in Butler, "Thirty Years of National Health Care," pp. 13-15.
84. Cooper, *Rationing Health Care*, p. 39.
85. Butler, "Thirty Years of National Health Care," p. 7.
86. Economic Models, Ltd., *The British Health Care System*, p. 85.
87. *British Medical Journal*, June 11, 1977, p. 1,531.
88. John Walsh, "Britain's National Health Service: The Doctor's Dilemmas," *Science*, Vol. 201, July, 1978, pp. 325-329.
89. Swartz, "The Infirmity of British Medicine," p. 38.
90. Cooper, *Rationing Health Care*, p. 39.
91. Economic Models, Ltd., *The British Health Care System*, p. 90.
92. *British Medical Journal*, December 6, 1975, p. 542.
93. John Roper, "N.H.S. in Crisis 3: Impossibility of Finding Money to Meet Demands," *The* (London) *Times*, August 11, 1978.
94. Cooper, *Rationing Health Care*, p. 39.
95. *Ibid.*
96. "Equal Care: The Decline of a Social Ideal," *The* (London) *Sunday Times*, May 13, 1973.
97. *Ibid.*
98. Studies show that elderly patients complain much less frequently than young patients. See Cooper, *Rationing Health Care*, p. 95.
99. Nicholas Bosanquet, "Immigrants and the N.H.S.," *New Society*, Vol. 17, July 1975, p. 130.
100. Economic Models, Ltd., *The British Health Care System*, Table 5.5, p. 88.
101. Quoted in Cooper, *Rationing Health Care*, p. 40.
102. "Diagnosis for a Cure: An Injection of Political Will."
103. Cooper, *Rationing Health Care*, p. 68.
104. *Ibid*, p. 40.
105. *Ibid*, p. 95.
106. Walsh, "Britain's National Health Service," p. 325.
107. Swartz, "The Infirmity of British Medicine," p. 33.
108. Quoted in Butler, "Thirty Years of National Health Care," p. 8.
109. Walsh, "Britain's National Health Service," p. 328. I have expressed these salaries in terms of U.S. currency using a conversion rate of £1 = $2.
110. *Ibid.*
111. *Ibid.*

112. See John Fisher, "If Britain's Health Care is So Bad, Why Do Patients Like It?" *Medical Economics,* August 21, 1978, p. 83.

113. Zachary Y. Dyckman, *A Study of Physicians' Fees: A Staff Report Prepared by the President's Council on Wage and Price Stability* (Washington, D.C.: Government Printing Office, 1978), p. 78.

114. Economic Models, Ltd., *The British Health Care System,* p. 88.

115. Based on information contained in Rudolf Klein, "Private Practice," *New Society,* Oct. 23, 1975, p. 215.

116. Swartz, "The Infirmity of British Medicine," p. 38.

117. *Ibid,* p. 33.

118. Anthony J. Culyer, "Health: The Social Cost of Doctors' Discretion," *New Society,* February 27, 1975, p. 518.

119. Powell, *The Politics of Medicine,* p. 36. (Emphasis added.)

120. *Report on Confidential Inquiries Into Maternal Deaths in England and Wales, 1967-9* (London: Her Majesty's Stationery Office, 1972).

121. *Report on an Inquiry into Maternal Deaths in Scotland, 1967-71.*

122. Cooper, *Rationing Health Care,* p. 103.

123. Swartz, "The Infirmity of British Medicine," pp. 37-38.

124. Derrick Henderson, "The British Triangle," *Private Practice,* April, 1978, p. 58.

125. Quoted in Butler, "Thirty Years of National Health Care," pp. 12-13.

126. "Higher Still and Higher," *The Economist,* October 14, 1978, p. 107.

127. For a brief history of the union movement among hospital workers, see David Widgery, "Unions and Strikes in the National Health Service in Britain," *International Journal of Health Services,* Vol. 6, No. 2, 1976.

128. Butler, "Thirty Years of National Health Care," p. 12.

129. *Daily Telegraph,* March 1, 1978. Reported in Butler, "Thirty Years of National Health Care," pp. 17-18.

130. *Daily Telegraph,* February 28, 1978. Reported in Butler, "Thirty Years of National Health Care," p. 18.

131. *Daily Telegraph,* March 9, 1978. Reported in Butler, "Thirty Years of National Health Care," p. 18.

132. *The* (London) *Times,* May 20, 1978. Reported in Butler, "Thirty Years of National Health Care," p. 18.

133. "Dirty Linen," *The Economist,* October 28, 1978, p. 20.

134. *On Call,* March 16, 1978.

135. Lejeune, "Out of the Window," p. 39. Some of the specific facts of this case have been disputed.

136. Economic Models, Ltd., *The British Health Care System,* pp. 113-114.

137. *Report of the Committee on Hospital Complaints Procedure* (Davis Committee) (London: Her Majesty's Stationery Office, 1973).

138. J. Leahy Taylor, "Malpractice in the United Kingdom," *International Journal of Health Services,* Vol. 6, No. 4, 1976, p. 629.

139. Economic Models, Ltd., *The British Health Care System,* p. 114.

140. Taylor, "Malpractice in the United Kingdom," p. 635.

141. *Ibid,* p. 636.

142. *Williams v. City of Detroit.* Michigan Circuit Court, Wayne County, Docket No. 182809, 1975.

143. Taylor, "Malpractice in the United Kingdom," p. 638.

144. *Ibid.*

145. Quoted in Paul F. Gemmill, *Britain's Search for Health* (Philadelphia: University of Pennsylvania Press, 1960), p. 20.

146. Culyer, *Need and the National Health Service,* p. 115.

147. Smith, "Verdict on N.H.S."

148. Ruth Levitt, *The Reorganized National Health Service* (London: Croom Helm, Ltd., 1976), p. 181.
149. Rozbicki, *Rationing British Health Care*, p. 16.
150. M. J. Buxton and R. E. Klein, "Distribution of Hospital Provision: Policy Themes and Resource Variations," *British Medical Journal*, February 8, 1975.
151. Michael Cooper and Anthony Culyer, "Equality in the N.H.S.: Intentions, Performance and Problems in Evaluation," in M.M. Houser, ed., *The Economics of Medical Care* (London: Allen and Unwin, 1972).
152. Cooper, *Rationing Health Care*, p. 67.
153. Peggy Nuttall, "The British National Health Service," *Nursing Outlook,* Vol. 25, No. 2, February, 1977, p. 100.
154. Economic Models, Ltd., *The British Health Care System*, p. 87.
155. Cooper, *Rationing Health Care*, p. 61.
156. *Ibid*, pp. 72-73.
157. R. J. Lavers and D. Whynes, "Hospital Productivity Trends in the Swinging Sixties," paper given at the Health Economists' Study Group Meeting in July, 1975. Reproduced in Culyer, *Need and the National Health Service*, p 74.
158. See Culyer, *Need and the National Health Service*, pp. 74-75.
159. Victor Fuchs, *Who Shall Live?* (New York: Basic Books, 1974), p. 98.
160. *Ibid.*
161. Paul T. Lahti, "Early Post-Operative Discharge of Patients from the Hospital," *Surgery*, 63, No. 3 (March 1968) pp. 410-415.
162. C. J. Roberts, "Implications of Shortening the Time Spent in Hospital," in *Health Care in a Changing Setting: the U.K. Experience,* CIBA Foundation Symposium, no. 43 (Amsterdam: Elsevier, 1976), p. 45.
163. Brian Abel-Smith, *Value for Money in Health Services* (New York: St. Martin's Press, 1976), p. 112.
164. *Ibid.*
165. Fuchs, *Who Shall Live?*, p. 99.
166. Cooper, *Rationing Health Care*, p. 55.
167. *Ibid*, pp. 55-56.
168. *Ibid*, p. 98.
169. See *The Report of a Sub-Committee of the Standing Maternity and Mid-wifery Advisory Committee* (London: Her Majesty's Stationery Office, 1970).
170. Cooper, *Rationing Health Care*, p. 101.
171. *Ibid*, p. 92.
172. *Ibid*, p. 93.
173. Rudolf Klein, "The Rise and Decline of Policy Analysis: The Strange Case of Health Policymaking in Britain," *Policy Analysis*, vol. 2, June, 1976.

Chapter 7
Rationing: Other N.H.S. Sectors

In addition to general practitioner and hospital services, the N.H.S. provides five other major types of services to British citizens: pharmaceutical services, general dental services, general ophthalmic services, community health services and "other" services. As Table 7-1 shows, the first four of these services have accounted for a declining portion of N.H.S. spending over the last decade. Between 1966 and 1976, spending on pharmaceutical services fell from 11.2 percent to 8.9 percent of N.H.S. spending. Spending on general dental services fell from 5.2 percent to 3.9 percent of total spending. In ophthalmic services, the drop was from 1.5 percent to 1.2 percent. In community health services, the share of total spending fell from 10.2 percent to 6.1 percent.

This decline is partly explained by a redefinition of N.H.S. spending categories in 1969. Probably a more basic reason for the decline is the introduction of *user charges* for certain types of dental, ophthalmic and pharmaceutical services. As we shall see, the existence of such charges has greatly reduced the rationing problem in these sectors of the N.H.S.

Community Health and "Other" Services

When the N.H.S. was being created, one of the most important acts taken was the nationalization of all British hospitals. This meant that most hospitals were taken out of the hands of local governments and placed under the control of Regional Hospital Boards. The local authorities (as local government units are collectively known), however, retained responsibility for environmental health and, over the years, began to assume more and more responsibilities in the personal health field.[1] Prior to 1974, these personal health services were generally referred to as *local health authority services*. After the 1974 reorganization of the N.H.S., however, most of the local authority services became classified under the heading of "community health services," and a few others (such as the ambulance service) became classified under the heading of "other" services.

Table 7-1

N.H.S. EXPENDITURE BY TYPE, SELECTED YEARS

(in percentages)

Year	Hospital Services	Pharmaceutical Services	General Medical Services	General Dental Services	General Ophthalmic Services	Local Authority Health	Other[1]	Total
1951	55.7	9.7	9.5	7.8	2.8	8.5	6.0	100.0
1955	57.2	9.5	10.2	6.3	2.5	8.9	5.4	100.0
1960	57.2	10.1	10.0	6.3	2.0	9.1	5.3	100.0
1965	60.4	11.1	7.8	5.1	1.6	10.3	3.7	100.0
1969[2]	63.1	10.4	8.0	4.9	1.5	7.8	4.3	100.0
1970	64.1	10.0	8.4	4.9	1.4	7.0	4.2	100.0
1971	65.3	9.8	8.1	4.9	1.3	7.0	3.6	100.0
1972	65.9	9.7	7.9	4.5	1.2	6.8	4.0	100.0
1973	66.2	9.4	7.4	4.4	1.1	6.9	4.6	100.0
1974[3]	67.0	8.7	6.5	4.3	1.0	5.7	6.8	100.0
1975	65.8	8.4	6.1	4.0	1.3	6.1	8.3	100.0
1976	63.0	8.9	6.1	3.9	1.2	6.1	10.8	100.0

1. Includes headquarters administration (RHAs, AHAs, Health Boards and Boards of Governors), central administration, ambulance services, mass radiography services, etc., and centrally financed items such as laboratory, vaccine and research and development costs, etc., not falling within the finance of any one service. Figures from 1974 are not strictly comparable with earlier years.

2. Change in definition of N.H.S. Certain local health authority services transferred from N.H.S. to Social Services.

3. Reorganization of N.H.S. Administration of certain N.H.S. community health services transferred from local authorities to new AHAs. School health services formerly administered by the Department of Education and Science also transferred to the N.H.S.

Source: Office of Health Economics, *The Cost of the N.H.S.*, OHE Briefing No. 7 (London: Office of Health Economics, October 1978), Table 2.

Despite the term "local," these services are no longer under the direct control of local governments. The 1974 reorganization scheme took them out of the hands of democratically elected local authorities and placed them under the control of Area Health Authorities. Local representatives still sit on the governing committees, however, and it is not clear that the reorganization has had any profound impact on the delivery of health services.[2]

Although this sector of the N.H.S. has received comparatively little attention from health economists and other researchers, it is an important one. It recently employed as many as 75,000 people in England and Wales, — including 1,500 doctors and dentists.[3] The personal health services offered include:

Ambulance
Health Centers
Health Visiting
Family Planning
Vaccination and Immunization
Other Preventive Care Facilities
Home Nursing and Midwifery

From an American perspective, British patients who have access to these services are in an enviable position. We have already mentioned the incredible number of ambulance rides taken by patients for non-emergency purposes. (This service, incidentally, cost the N.H.S. approximately $233 million in 1976.[4]) In addition, nearly eight million house calls were made in 1976 by home nurses and health visitors. Eight million is the equivalent of 14 percent of the British population and perhaps one-half of all British homes. The purpose of these visits ranged from care for post-operative and chronically-ill patients to prenatal and infant care, as well as family planning and nutrition. In addition, over 1.3 million visits were made to patients' homes by chiropodists. About 172,000 people were served in their homes by the "meals on wheels" program, and about 653,000 elderly, chronically ill, and handicapped patients received "home help service" for house alterations, personal appliances (telephones, televisions and radios) and other arrangements that permitted them to remain out of hospitals.[5]

While Americans may be envious of the ability to receive such services, they should be forewarned of the gloomy side of the picture. For one thing, with local authority services free to the user, the quantity demanded of such services naturally exceeds the quantity being supplied. So invariably a shortage of local authority services is perceived. For another, while the quantity of such services appears large, their quality and the wisdom of allocating funds in this way are open to considerable doubt.

One of the biggest problems in the N.H.S. hospital sector is the number of beds being occupied by the chronic and long-term sick — people who are in need of care but not necessarily in need of *hospital* care. In the previous chapter we pointed out that, while thousands of urgent patients are on hospital waiting lists, about 25 percent of all acute hospital beds are occupied by people who do not need to be there. These are mainly patients whose presence in the hospital is due to the inadequacies of care in the community in which they live.[6] In 1971, a British Medical Association Panel reported on the seriousness of the problem:

> There is a delay in transferring geriatric cases from acute hospital beds, thus creating delays in acute admissions. The evidence is that this is almost entirely due to insufficient local authority accommodation and other suitable community care, meaning a delay in discharge from geriatric hospitals.[7]

Compared to the United States, Britain has very few nursing homes.[8] And it appears that home visiting is simply an inadequate alternative to institution-based care for many of the elderly and the chronically ill. But it is wasteful and inefficient to keep such patients in hospitals. Hospitals are ideally designed for intensive treatment administered to short-term-stay patients. As one study has concluded:

> There would be scope for considerable savings if a large portion of hospitalized cases could, without detriment to the patient, be treated outside the hospital. If that were the case, higher priority for investment in community-based facilities such as health centers and residential accommodation for the elderly would be indicated on both economic and social grounds.[9]

Should the N.H.S. fail to make such changes, the problem will become increasingly aggravated. If present trends continue, according to two health experts, by 1992, 93.7 percent of all nonmaternity beds available for women and 73.5 percent of all beds available for men will be filled with old age pensioners.[10]

Local health authorities are also responsible for vaccination and immunization against certain infectious diseases, particularly childhood diseases. These vaccinations are carried out in local authority health clinics or by arrangements with general practitioners. The service, however, leaves much to be desired. As Table 7-2 shows, over the last decade there has been a decline in the percentage of children vaccinated against every major childhood disease. The difference between British medical care and American medical care in this area is vividly expressed in the comments of Dr. Nicholas P. Krikes, President of the California Medical Association and a recent visitor to England.

In this town of High Wycombe — with no appreciable slums, excellent light industry and in general a very beautiful town — there were 245 cases of measles last year. If we had 245 cases of measles in my city, which has three times the population of High Wycombe, there would be considerable consternation and corrective effort.[11]

Table 7-2

PREVENTIVE MEDICINE: VACCINATION

	Percentages and thousands							
	1961	1966	1971	1972	1973	1974	1975	1976
Children born in preceding calendar year who were vaccinated by end of year stated (percentages):								
Diphtheria	—	73	65	65	64	57	57	56
Whooping Cough	—	72	64	63	61	51	32	32
Poliomyelitis	—	69	64	64	62	57	57	56
Tetanus	—	72	65	65	63	57	57	56
Number of people under age 16 who were vaccinated in the year (thousands):								
Measles	—	—	594	581	521	405	350	367
Rubella	—	—	439	322	295	288	298	334
Number of people who were vaccinated in the year (thousands):								
Tuberculosis	611	564	659	645	679	646	684	730

Source: Department of Health and Social Security, *Social Trends* (London: Her Majesty's Stationery Office, 1977), p. 148.

As in other areas of the health service, inequalities in the availability of treatment are widespread. Table 7-3 shows the distribution of spending on community health services by health region. In general, community health and other services are distributed more equally than hospital services, but less equally than the general practitioner services.[12]

Table 7-3

COMMUNITY HEALTH AND "OTHER" SERVICES
EXPENDITURE PER CAPITA BY REGION
Year Ended March 1976[1]

	Population All Ages	Community Health Services Per Capita	Other Services Per Capita
ENGLAND	46,435	5.60	2.84
Northern	3,125	5.33	2.91
Yorkshire	3,582	4.85	2.63
Trent	4,545	5.15	2.37
East Anglia	1,781	4.59	2.71
N.W. Thames	3,470	6.05	3.09
N.E. Thames	3,714	6.27	2.82
S.E. Thames	3,599	6.06	3.04
S.W. Thames	2,883	6.30	3.48
Wessex	2,640	5.29	2.38
Oxford	2,198	6.12	2.85
Southwestern	3,148	5.08	3.03
West Midlands	5,176	5.56	2.64
Mersey	2,501	5.53	3.04
North Western	4,074	5.99	2.88

1. Excluding hospitals directly administered by the Department of Health and Social Security, and supply and repair of artificial limbs and appliances.
Source: Department of Health and Social Security, *Health and Personal Social Services Statistics for England*, 1977 (London: Her Majesty's Stationery Office), Table 2.7, p. 22.

General Dental Services

One of the major concerns of the founding fathers of the N.H.S. was the state of dental health in the British population. Much of the problem, however, appeared to be cultural and not economic. As one observer put it, "the British people are astonishingly neglectful of their teeth."[13] Before the N.H.S. was established, for example, many of the insured working population were entitled to dental care under the national health insurance scheme then in force. Yet only 6 percent of those insured claimed dental benefits.[14]

During World War II, a government Committee on Dental Services reported on the poor state of dental health, and called for a substantial increase in the number of dentists once the N.H.S. was underway.[15] Yet in 1972, the number of dentists per capita in England was smaller than it was in 1949.[16] The state of dental health has apparently not fared much better. Over a decade after the beginning of the N.H.S., a British journalist reported that "in one county it was recently discovered that half the school pupils did not even have a toothbrush. Dental decay has approximately doubled among children in the last ten years."[17] A more recent study found that 90 percent of the nondenture wearers in Darlington and Salisbury needed dental treatment. Over 70 percent needed periodental treatment (for inflamation of the gum leading to the loss of teeth), and 75 percent had decayed teeth. Even so, about 40 percent of those examined thought they required no treatment at all.[18]

Nonetheless, the fact that demand for dental services is high (much higher than the N.H.S. was prepared to meet) while the "price" is zero became apparent very quickly in 1948. Eight months after the N.H.S. scheme was launched, a supplementary estimate put before Parliament concluded that the required budget for dental services would be three times the original projection.[19]

Two methods are now used by the N.H.S. to control the demand for dental services. One method, used from the beginning of the health services, is the Central Dental Estimates Board. All treatment outside of minor dental work must have the prior approval of this board if the treatment is to be covered by the N.H.S. Many dental services that would be considered "necessary" under most U.S. private health insurance policies are often considered "luxuries" by the Estimates Board, and are consequently denied coverage. The Estimates Board, moreover, is yet another instance of a top-heavy beauraucracy within the N.H.S. As early as 1948, there was one board member for every ten dentists.[20]

Another way in which the demand for dental services is discouraged is through *user fees*. Although charging a fee to patients for dental services was obhorent to the socialist leaders of the Labour Party, they introduced such fees in 1951 to stem the enormous drain the dental service was placing on the N.H.S. budget. The initial fees were only for dentures, and represented about one-half their actual cost. In 1952, user fees were extended (subject to a £1 maximum) to all dental services.[21] The effect on demand was substantial. By 1952, the demand for dentures alone had decreased by 60 percent from the previous year.[22]

In 1971, a new form of cost-related dental charge was introduced. Patients were required to pay one-half the cost of treatment up to a maximum of £10. Certain routine services such as a clinical examination, however, were excluded from the charge. In addition, persons under 21 years of age, expectant mothers, and low-income individuals were made exempt from user charges.[23] In 1976, the N.H.S. spent almost $95 million subsidizing dentures.[24]

Like the general practitioner, the dentist practicing in the N.H.S. is not an employee of the state. Instead he is an independent contractor who performs certain services for the state in return for negotiated fees. Almost from the beginning of the N.H.S., these fees have been a source of great bitterness among Britain's dentists. In 1977, the average dentist earned less than $14,000 (before taxes) from his N.H.S. work. Yet it can cost a dentist up to $50,000 to set up his practice.[25]

As a result of continuing disputes (mainly over pay), a situation has recently developed in the dental service that can only be described as open revolt. Apparently, Britain's dentists are simply opting out of the N.H.S. in increasing numbers. In 1978, the (London) *Daily Mail* described the conditions this way:

> The charges for what started 30 years ago as a completely free service seem to be going up by the visit. And increasingly, N.H.S. patients are finding that they can't get treated at all.
>
> Try asking today for a crown or a bridge, or a denture repair, and you may well be told that unless you are prepared to pay for treatment you had better go somewhere else.
>
> An ever-growing number of Britain's 15,000 practicing dentists are now refusing to provide certain treatment on the N.H.S. — and at least a third of them will only take you as a new patient if you agree to pay in full under a completely private arrangement.[26]

Moreover, *The* (London) *Times* recently reported that there are entire areas of Britain "where dentists no longer accept any N.H.S. patients and intend to keep it that way."[27]

Those dentists who *do* remain within the N.H.S. will undoubtedly be distributed unequally across the various health regions. As Table 7-4 shows, dentists are distributed more unequally than general practitioners, and the inequality in the distribution has worsened over time. Moreover, those health regions that are more endowed with other health services also tend to be more endowed with dentists.[28]

Ophthalmic Services

Like the dental services furnished by the newborn N.H.S., the

Table 7-4

GENERAL DENTAL PRACTITIONERS PER 10,000 POPULATION
BY HEALTH REGION, 1977

Health Region	No. of Dentists Per 10,000 Population
ENGLAND	2.55
Northern	1.84
Yorkshire	2.18
Trent	1.88
East Anglia	2.20
N.W. Thames	4.01
N.E. Thames	2.77
S.E. Thames	2.91
S.W. Thames	3.61
Wessex	2.72
Oxford	2.51
South Western	2.97
West Midlands	2.10
Mersey	2.44
North Western	2.12
WALES	2.09
SCOTLAND	2.33
N. IRELAND	2.27
UNITED KINGDOM	2.50

Source: *Royal Commission on the National Health Service Report* (Merrison Report) (London: Her Majesty's Stationery Office, 1979), Table 3.2, p. 16.

ophthalmic services witnessed a surge in demand that went well beyond initial predictions. Three million pairs of eyeglasses had been made available for the first year of the N.H.S.; two million were gone after the first eight weeks. When the supplementary estimate was placed before Parliament eight months after the scheme had begun, the new budget requirement for the ophthalmic service was over six times the original budget! By 1951, 17 million pairs of spectacles had been issued.[29]

There is also evidence that a great deal of waste took place in the early years. In 1950, for example, the number of spectacles supplied was nearly 70 percent greater than the number of sight tests carried out. The Labour Government responded in the same way it had to the demand for dentures — with user charges. In 1951, consumers were charged for spectacles at the rate of £1 per pair, plus the actual cost of the frame. The response was once again dramatic. The number of spectacles dropped by 60 percent from 1950 to 1952, while the number of sight tests fell by 25 percent.[30] To further eliminate waste, patients were charged the *whole cost* of eyeglasses, plus a dispensing fee of £1 4s if replacements were requested because of the patients' lack of care.[31]

Under the N.H.S., ophthalmic medical practitioners and ophthalmic opticians may test sight and prescribe glasses, while ophthalmic opticians and dispensing opticians supply glasses to prescription. Both practitioners and opticians are independent contractors and are paid negotiated fees for sight tests. Fees are also paid by the N.H.S. for the supply of glasses. Diagnosis and specialist treatment of eye conditions are available under the Hospital Eye Service.[32]

Today, a range of prices exist for N.H.S. frames. Although privately manufactured frames are more expensive, they are far more popular. It is significant that while the total N.H.S. spending on ophthalmic services in 1968 was £16 million, £26 million was spent by patients on private frames, tests and lenses.[33] Moreover, the number of spectacles supplied by the N.H.S. has declined in recent years. In 1976, for example, the number of N.H.S. spectacles supplied dropped from 6.2 million pairs to 5.9 million.[34] Like dental services, then, it appears that ophthalmic services are becoming increasingly private. Nonetheless, in 1976, the N.H.S. spent about $48 million giving people "free" eyesight tests.[35]

Pharmaceutical Services

On the average, British citizens seem to enjoy taking drugs. Every tenth night's sleep in Britain is drug-induced. Nineteen percent of all British women and nine percent of all men are taking tranquillizers during the course of any one year. And according to one authority, "it is likely that by 1990 nearly every individual will be taking psychotropic medicines either continuously or at intervals."[36]

The central financial problem in the pharmaceutical service is precisely the same as it is in the dental and ophthalmic services: "the payer (the state) is a separate person from the orderer (the prescribing doctor) and the consumer (the patient)."[37] Under these circumstances, all the principal parties to drug consumption decisions have an incentive to spend a great deal of the taxpayer's money. Enoch Powell explains why:

> In the supply of drugs outside the hospitals, the state confronts an array of parties all severally interested in maximizing the value of the volume of the drugs supplied. The general practitioner, on behalf of his patient, and sometimes

in deference to his patient, is interested in prescribing the most efficacious medicines and is insulated from consideration of cost. The patient, equally insulated from consideration of cost, is naturally concerned to get the most efficacious medicines and is equally naturally disposed to gauge efficacy by cost and novelty — the two are closely connected. The manufacturers and patentees of the medicines are naturally concerned to sell as much as possible of the most expensive of these wares and to do so at as high a price as possible; and since price is not here performing its function of balancing supply and demand, there is no point . . . beyond which increase of the price reduces the return. Finally, the distributors and dispensers of medicines — the pharmacists — are naturally interested in maximizing the value and volume of their turn-over . . .

The 'budget' for the pharmaceutical service is not a budget in the ordinary sense of so much and no more. It is only a hopeful guess at how much others are going to spend. The long and arduous story of drugs and the state is the story of the various attempts of the state to 'get at' the parties to the drug transaction in spite of its own lack of direct powers.[38]

That story begins with the beginning of the N.H.S. At that time it was estimated that patients would require 140 million prescriptions per year. But like spectacles and dentures, the flood of actual prescriptions left original predictions shattered in its wake. In the first nine months of N.H.S. operation, prescriptions were running at an annual rate of 190 million, and the original budget for the pharmaceutical service was increased by 40 percent.[39] The event provoked Aneurin Bevan's famous tirade about "cascades of medicine pouring down British throats."[40]

The government's response was, of course, predictable. In 1952, a flat-rate user charge of one shilling per prescription was introduced. The number of prescriptions dropped by 8 million that year, even though the charge was not introduced until June. User charges were raised to one shilling per item — making them equal to about 20 percent of the average cost of a prescription — in December of 1956. The following year, the number of prescriptions fell by 22 million.[41]

In 1961, charges were again raised to equal about 20 percent of the then higher average cost of prescriptions. But in 1965, the Labour Party abolished user charges for prescriptions altogether. The results were dramatic! Within three years the number of prescriptions had risen 30 percent. Charges were reintroduced in 1968, leading to a ten percent drop in the number of prescriptions over the next two years.[42]This rollercoaster ride of prescriptions is depicted in Figure 7-1.

Currently, user charges continue to reflect about 20 percent of the actual cost of prescriptions. A number of people are exempt from such charges, however. These include children, the elderly and low-income persons. The exemptions appear to be important. Out of 248 million prescriptions dispensed in 1970/71, 133 million (or 54 percent) were dispensed to exempt people.[43]

The health service has also taken a number of steps to inhibit the prescription proclivities of general practitioners. One step consists of a great deal of exhortation. According to Powell, the idea is to

try to persuade the prescriber to behave voluntarily as it is supposed he would behave if he and his patient had to have regard to the cost of what he prescribes. The attempt shares the weakness of all policies that assume the fulfillment of an unfulfilled condition. In pursuit of it doctors have been bombarded with information about the comparative cost of drugs, advised on equivalents or near-equivalents, urged to prefer non-proprietary to proprietary preparations where possible, coached and lectured on how to write a non-proprietary prescription (instead of an easy, catchy brand name), stiffened to resist the visual and personal blandishments of the advertisers and salesmen of proprietary medicines — and all to little purpose.[44]

Other steps have been to much more purpose. General practitioners whose prescription policies are out of line with those of other doctors in their area may be called to task for excessive prescribing by the Medical Practices Committee. In extreme cases, the doctor may actually be fined.[45] One of the problems with such a policy is that prescribing practices vary considerably from region to region.[46] Even within the hospital sector, for example, drug expenditure per patient varies as much as 40 percent among health regions.[47] So a doctor's prescriptions may be out of line with the prescribing policies of his area merely because he is matching the standard of excellence met in some other area, but not achieved in his own. In addition, doctors may have very different types of patients with different types of medical needs on their lists. Ann Cartwright relates the case of a

Figure 7-1

PHARMACEUTICAL PRESCRIPTIONS IN THE N.H.S.

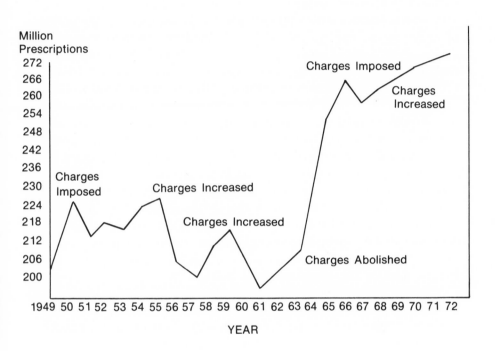

Source: Economic Models, Ltd., *The British Health Care System* (Chicago: American Medical Association, 1976), Figure 7.12, p. 153. Reprinted with permission of the American Medical Association.

doctor who had an unusually high number of elderly chronics on his patient list. After being hassled about his prescribing policies, he asked all the chronic patients who lived more than a mile from his office to leave his list.[48] Although Cartwright discovered a number of doctors who believed that the government's policy was injurious to the health of their patients, Professor Dennis Lees believes the problem is much less serious today.[49]

Another policy which inhibits general practitioners is the policy of reserving the right to prescribe more modern and more expensive drugs to the hospital sector, over which the N.H.S. has more direct control.[50] In Britain, general practitioners typically prescribe from a list of about 3,000 medicines, although the number is 7,500 in Germany, 12,000 in Italy and perhaps even higher in the U.S.[51]

A final method of controlling drug costs in the N.H.S. consists of pressuring the drug companies who supply them to keep prices down. A number of observers have claimed that the N.H.S. enjoys the conditions of *monopsony* with respect to the pharmaceutical market.[52] Monopsony is a market in which there is a single buyer, and is often contrasted with monopoly — a market in which there is a single seller. Just as a monopolist (single seller) is thought to be able to exploit consumers, so a monopsonist (single buyer) is thought to be able to exploit producers and sellers. This, it is alledged, is precisely what the N.H.S. does in the pharmaceutical market.

Enoch Powell denies that the N.H.S. possesses any significant monopsony power. Nonetheless, he concedes that the state's position as the sole buyer (or almost the sole buyer) of ethical drugs creates on the part of the sellers a "countervailing political fear."[53] Why such fear should arise is illustrated by the events that took place in 1961. In that year a number of hospitals reported that they were being offered drugs by importers at prices far below those prevailing in current contracts. The importers, it seems, were offering drugs from Italy (which did not allow patents on drugs), and from certain communist countries (which do not recognize Western patents at all). Normally, Britain is obliged to respect international patents. But a special provision of the Patents Act allows the purchase of goods sold without license from the patentee "for the service of the Crown." In this case, a sum may be paid to the patentee. But the sum may be determined by the British government, rather than through bargaining with the patentee. From 1961 through 1965, the N.H.S. purchased through non-licensed sellers on the basis of this special provision of the Patents Act. After 1965, it resumed its purchases from licensed sellers, but only at what has been described as "acceptable prices."[54]

A number of studies have shown that the prices paid by the N.H.S. are considerably lower than the prices paid in other countries for the same drugs. The results of one of these studies are reproduced in Table 7-5. The conclusions of all such studies are somewhat suspect. Like all international comparisons, these studies face the tough problems of coping with international exchange rates. In addition, drug prices may legitimately differ because of differences in transportation costs and other costs. Nonetheless, there is plenty of indication that, when all adjustments are made, the British pay less for drugs than the citizens of other countries.

Table 7-5

DIFFERENCES BETWEEN AVERAGE OVERSEAS PRICES AND U.K. PRICES FOR PHARMACEUTICALS

Percent of U.K. price based on currency exchange rates.

$$\frac{Overseas\ Average\ Price - U.K.\ Average\ Price}{U.K.\ average\ price} \times 100$$

Country	U.K. weighted		Overseas weighted	
	1964	1970	1964	1970
Belgium	—	+19	—	+33
Finland	—	+20	—	+21
France	− 5	+ 8	− 9	+10
Germany	+15	+27	− 2	+35
Italy	+25	+97	+24	+80
Japan	—	+60	—	−55
Spain	+ 4	+14	− 3	+31
Turkey	—	+27	—	+30

Note: "Minus" signs indicate the percentage by which the overseas market is cheaper than in the United Kingdom; "plus" signs indicate the percentage by which it is more expensive.

Source: M.H. and A.J. Cooper, *International Price Comparisons* (a study of the prices of pharmaceuticals in the United Kingdom and eight other countries) (London: NEDO, 1972), pp. 5 and 6. Reproduced by permission of Her Majesty's Stationery office.

What is not clear is *why* the British pay less. A possible reason is the monopsony power of the N.H.S. discussed above. Yet if monopsony power accounts for lower drug prices, it has not produced lower rates of return for drug manufacturers. The average rate of return on capital for the pharmaceutical industry is about 25 percent, compared to about 14 percent for all manufacturing concerns.[55] These numbers are quite comparable to the rates of return that prevail in the United States.[56]

Another possible explanation for low drug prices in Britain is the fact that fewer *different* types of drugs are sold there. This means inventory and handling costs to the suppliers are probably lower than in other countries. Still another contributing factor may be the lower promotional costs incurred in Britain. In 1971, pharmaceutical companies spent an average of $5,000 per doctor promoting drugs in the United States.[57] Yet in Britain in 1974, advertising expenditure per doctor was less than half (£650) that amount.[58] Moreover, 1976 legislation in Britain actually prohibits what is described as "wasteful" advertising practices.[59]

Nonetheless, the N.H.S. spends an enormous amount of money each year subsidizing the consumption of pharmaceuticals, many of which are only marginally related to health. For example, in 1975 the N.H.S. spent $9 million subsidizing "free" contraceptives, over $12 million on sleeping pills, almost $21 million on tranquilizers and sedatives, $11 million on cough medicine, and almost $4 million on vitamins.[60] These numbers appear especially incredible when it is realized that *up to one-third of all patients do not take the prescriptions they receive.*[61]

Footnotes

1. Economic Models, Ltd., *The British Health Care System* (Chicago: American Medical Association, 1976), p. 116.
2. Michael Cooper, *Rationing Health Care* (New York: Halsted Press, 1975), p. 73.
3. Economic Models, Ltd., *The British Health Care System*, p. 116.
4. Based on estimates in Office of Health Economics, *OHE Briefing*, No. 7, (London: OHE, 1978).
5. See Department of Health and Social Security, *Health and Personal Social Services Statistics for England*, 1977.
6. Economic Models, Ltd., *The British Health Care System*, p. 110.
7. "Gaps in Medical Care — Report of an Inquiry by Special Panel Appointed by the Board of Science and Education of the B.M.A.," *British Medical Journal Supplement*, May 8, 1971, p. 89.
8. Derek Robinson, "Primary Medical Practice in the United Kingdom and in the United States," *The New England Journal of Medicine*, 297, July 28, 1977, p. 190.
9. Economic Models, Ltd., *The British Health Care System*, p. 111.
10. R. Klein and J. Ashley, "Old Age Health," *New Society*, January 6, 1972.
11. Nicholas P. Krikes, "Myths of the British National Health Service: An Eyewitness Account," reprinted in *Vital Speeches*, February 1, 1978, p. 246.
12. See Anthony Culyer, *Need and the National Health Service* (Totowa, New Jersey: Rowman and Littlefield, 1976), Table 9.1, p. 114.
13. Colm Brogan, "Shortages as Seen by a Journalist", in Helmut Schoek, ed., *Financing Medical Care: An Appraisal of Foreign Programs* (Caldwell, Idaho: Caxton Printers, Ltd., 1962), p. 59.
14. Ruth Levitt, *The Reorganized National Health Service* (London: Croom Helm, Ltd., 1976), p. 109.
15. Mathew Lynch and Stanley Raphael, *Medicine and the State* (Oak Brook, Illinois: Association of American Physicians and Surgeons, 1973), p. 180.
16. Economic Models, Ltd., *The British Health Care System*, p. 106.
17. Brogan, "Shortages As Seen by a Journalist," p. 109.
18. J.S. Bulman, N.D. Richards, G.L. Slock and A.J. Willcocks, *Demand and Need for Dental Care* (Oxford: Nuffield Provincial Hospitals Trust, 1968).
19. Lynch and Raphael, *Medicine and the State*, p. 179.
20. *Ibid*, p. 181.
21. Economic Models, Ltd., *The British Health Care System*, p. 107.
22. *Ibid.*
23. *Ibid.*
24. *Health and Personal Social Services Statistics*, p. 90.
25. Stuart Butler, "Thirty Years of National Health Care: A Review of the British Experience" (Washington, D.C.: The Heritage Foundation, 1978), p. 9.
26. Quoted in Butler, "Thirty Years of National Health Care," p. 9.
27. "Dentists Asked to State if Treatment is Private," *The* (London) *Times*, June 14, 1978.
28. Economic Models, Ltd., *The British Health Care System*, p. 139.
29. Lynch and Raphael, *Medicine and the State*, p. 179.
30. Economic Models, Ltd., *The British Health Care System*, p. 107.
31. Lynch and Raphael, *Medicine and the State,* p. 138. Charges were instituted from the beginning for the replacement of dentures in cases where "carelessness" was the cause of damage or loss.
32. Economic Models, Ltd., *The British Health Care System*, pp. 107-8.
33. Office of Health Economics, *Ophthalmic Service* (London: Office of Health Economics, 1970).
34. Office of Health Economics, *OHE Briefing*, No. 7.

35. *Ibid.*
36. Cooper, *Rationing Health Care*, p. 105.
37. Enoch Powell, *Medicine and Politics: 1975 and After* (New York: Pitman, 1976), p. 64.
38. *Ibid*, pp. 59-60.
39. Lynch and Raphael, *Medicine and the State*, p. 179.
40. Quoted in Powell, *Medicine and Politics*, p. 61.
41. Lynch and Raphael, *Medicine and the State*, pp. 184-5.
42. Economic Models, Ltd., *The British Health Care System*, p. 106.
43. *Ibid.*
44. Powell, *Medicine and Politics*, p. 63.
45. M.F. Cuthbert, J.P. Griffin, and W.H.W. Inman, "The United Kingdom," in William Wardell, ed., *Controlling the Use of Therapeutic Drugs* (Washington, D.C.: American Enterprise Institute, 1978), pp. 133-4.
46. Powell, *Medicine and Politics*, p. 62.
47. Cooper, *Rationing Health Care*, p. 66.
48. Ann Cartwright, *Patients and Their Doctors* (London: Routledge and Kegan Paul, 1967), p. 59.
49. Dennis Lee, "Economics and Non-economics of Health Services, *Three Banks Review,* 110, June, 1976, p. 19.
50. Cuthbert, *et. al.*, "The United Kingdom," p. 133.
51. Organization for Economic Cooperation and Development, *Public Expenditure on Health* (Paris: OECD, 1977), p. 82.
52. See, for example, Alan Maynard, "Medical Care in the European Community," *New Society*, August 28, 1975.
53. Powell, *Medicine and Politics*, p. 64.
54. *Ibid*, pp. 65-6.
55. Levitt, *The Reorganized National Health Service*, p. 122.
56. Reported rates of return in the drug industry tend to be biased upward because the drug industry's heavy investment in research and development is not capitalized as is investment in physical capital. See Victor Fuchs, *Who Shall Live?* (New York: Basic Books, 1974), p. 121.
57. Abel-Smith, *Value for Money in Health Services*, p. 83.
58. OECD, *Public Expenditure on Health*, p. 80.
59. The regulation was included in the Voluntary Price Regulation Scheme (VPRS).
60. *Health and Personal Social Services Statistics*, pp. 113-6.
61. Cooper, *Rationing Health Care*, p. 102.

Chapter 8
The Trend Toward Private Care

In 1978, over 600,000 people were waiting to get into British hospitals. Many had been waiting for months and years, and an astonishing number were classified as "urgent" cases. Those who received treatment often did so in worn-out buildings with inadequate staffs in a health service whose sagging quality is now openly discussed in the British press.

That same year, a great many British patients found a better way. Although they had paid taxes to help finance the $16 billion the health service spent on "free" medical care,[1] they shelled out another $320 million for private health care.[2] About 2.5 million of them purchased private health insurance, either as individuals or through employer-financed group policies.[3] Since 1970, the amount spent on private medical services has been increasing at about eight percent per year in real terms. Over the last decade, the number of people covered by group health insurance policies has nearly doubled.[4] And by 1979, it was estimated that nearly four million people — over seven percent of Britain's population — had acquired some form of private health insurance.[5]

Private medical care in Britain is often as expensive as it is in the United States. So why are so many British citizens willing to pay for services that are theoretically made available for "free" by the state? An analogous question is: why are many middle-income American families willing to turn down "free" public education and spend up to $5,000 per year to send their children to private schools? The analogy fits fairly closely. Over 4 percent of U.S. school children attend private schools, and the boom in private school enrollment over the decade of the 1970s parallels the boom in private health insurance policies in Britain.[6]

In both cases, the existence of an active private market is amazing, because the price people pay for the private service does not merely reflect the value that people place on that service. It reflects the value they place on that service *given that state-provided service is available at no cost to the user.* Put another way, the price of private service reflects the value people place on that service *minus* the value they place on the state-provided alternative. If people are willing to pay for private medical care in Britain and private schooling in the U.S., clearly they must perceive the differential value between private and public services to be worth the price.

General Practitioners

All general practitioners in the N.H.S. system are free to have private patients, and most of them do. A recent survey revealed that only 38 percent of G.P.s had no private patients. About 5 percent have more than 100 private patients.[7] Under ten percent of Britain's general practitioners are engaged *exclusively* in private practice and operate outside the N.H.S.[8] Most of those G.P.s who have a large number of private patients are practicing in the comparatively affluent south of England.[9] It appears that G.P.s with as many as 50 to 100 private patients can earn as much from their private patients as they receive for treating 1,500 N.H.S. patients.[10]

It is estimated that between one and two percent of all adults see general practitioners as private patients. Many of these people, however, also see general practitioners as N.H.S. patients. And less than five percent of private health insurance subscribers in 1970 opted for general practice benefits.[11] Part of the explanation may be that private patients are not permitted to take advantage of the approximately 80 percent discount available to N.H.S. patients on prescriptions. In addition, it appears that many patients opt for N.H.S. care when their ailments are minor, and for private care when their conditions are more serious. As one general practitioner explained:

> Some people call me privately for anything they're worried about, and go to the Health Service for minor things. A family·called me in when a child had spots and a temperature. I explained it was chickenpox and nothing to worry about. When other children came out in a rash, they called the Health Service doctor. Then other N.H.S. patients come to me and say "I've seen [a Health Service doctor]; he gave me this prescription; would you copy it out?"; or, "I'm having a threatened miscarriage. I've seen [a Health Service doctor]. Please will you come and give the injections?"[12]

It might seem strange that a patient would call on a private doctor to fill out a prescription. But a recent study by the British Pharmaceutical Society found that less than 73 percent of the prescriptions surveyed had "adequate prescription details." It appears that one out of every ten prescriptions is filled out by someone other than the doctor — often by a receptionist — and merely signed by the doctor. Moreover, of those filled out by "others," 32 percent had no instructions on when and how to take the medicine.[13]

In general, patients who see doctors privately appear to believe that they receive a better quality of medical care than they receive as N.H.S. patients. Many also believe that private doctors can avoid delays in getting them into the hospital. Some elderly patients merely continued the private arrangements they had with their doctors before the N.H.S. was founded. And some middle-class patients apparently feel guilty about taking up the time of hurried, over-worked N.H.S. doctors.[14]

Surprisingly, a great many G.P.s are not enthusiastic about private patients. One early study found that about one-half the doctors surveyed discouraged private patients, or preferred not to have them. The reasons given for disliking private patients were that they were snobbish, inconsiderate, and "unable to accept a reasonable doctor-patient relationship." However, another one-third of those surveyed — presumably including the more successful doctors — liked having private patients.[15]

In general, then, private medical care exists very much on the periphery of the market for general practitioner services. It is important only to a small percentage of patients, and the attitudes of general practitioners are mixed. Things are much different in the hospital sector.

N.H.S. Hospitals

One of the most remarkable features of the N.H.S. hospital sector is the existence of private, or "pay beds," in N.H.S. hospitals. The pay beds have been a thorn in the side of socialist ideologues from the beginning. But their existence was part of an historic compromise between Aneurin Bevan and the hospital doctors — a compromise that won the consultants' consent to the formation of the Health Service.

Prior to 1948, many leading consultants practicing in (voluntary) teaching hospitals were not paid for their work. Their income came exclusively from private practice. Bevan knew that many of these doctors would be unwilling to accept full-time, salaried employment with the N.H.S. So Bevan agreed that, when these hospitals were nationalized, a small number of beds would be set aside for private practice, and consultants would have the option of taking part-time contracts, allowing them the freedom to treat some patients private-ly.[16]

To the hospital consultants, this compromise was on the order of a contract. But subsequent Labour Governments have increasingly shown a willingness to renege. As Figure 8-1 shows, the percentage of private beds in N.H.S. hospitals has been substantially reduced each time the Labour Party was in power. The most recent Labour Government came to power on a campaign pledge to eliminate private beds in N.H.S. hospitals altogether. What is more, once in office, Labour Party officials apparently planned to go further — to abolish private medicine in Britain.

In 1975, the Labour Government, under Prime Minister Harold Wilson, apparently planned not only to eliminate N.H.S. pay beds, but also to make it virtually impossible to build any significant number of private hospitals to replace the N.H.S. private beds. Moreover, a government memorandum leaked to the medical press outlined a scheme to relocate all general practitioners into government operated health centers, and then to prohibit the G.P.s from seeing private patients in these centers. All of this helped provoke a consultant's "slowdown" in mid-1975. The Wilson government promptly denied that it had any intentions of destroying private medicine.[17]

Much of the impetus to do away with pay beds comes from the more militant, left-wing segments of the Labour Party, including the hospital workers unions. The unions have long been critical of what is called a "dual" system of health care. They attack the pay beds as fostering "elitism" and "line-jumping."[18] No doubt many union members perceive that they have no economic stake in the pay beds. The nurses and staff who attend private patients receive no extra income for doing so. Only the consultant receives a private fee.[19]

This perception is not quite correct, however. As Table 8-1 shows, income to the N.H.S. from pay beds is not insignificant. Private patients are charged fees for their rooms and other services — fees which are comparable to those charged by private hospitals and nursing homes.[20] In 1976/77, for example, income to the N.H.S. from pay beds totalled £32 million. This is income added to the N.H.S. budget out of which wages and salaries are paid.

The substantial income from pay beds may account for the reluctance of even Labour governments to abolish them. Another reason may be that "many politicians and members of 'The Establishment' do not use the N.H.S. for routine treatment."[21]

Figure 8-1

PAY BEDS IN THE N.H.S.

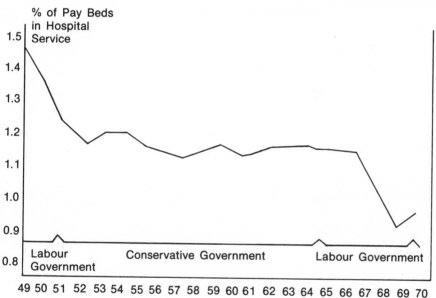

YEAR

Source: Economic Models Ltd., *The British Health Care System* (Chicago: The American Medical Association, 1976), Table 7.10, p. 148.

Table 8-1
INCOME FROM "PAY BEDS"

Year	£ million
1966/67	8
1967/68	8
1968/69	9
1969/70	11
1970/71	11
1971/72	13
1972/73	16
1973/74	19
1974/75	20
1975/76	25
1976/77	32

Note: Includes amenity beds (private rooms for N.H.S. patients), but the income from these is too small to alter figures significantly.

Source: Stuart Butler, "Thirty Years of National Health Care: A Review of the British Experience" (Washington, D.C.: Heritage Foundation, 1978), p. 16.

Why is it that each year tens of thousands of British citizens are willing to pay (either directly or indirectly through insurance premiums) fees to consultants and to the N.H.S. for private medical care? There seem to be four reasons: (1) they believe they get a better quality of medical care; (2) in case of surgery, they are able to choose which doctor will actually do the operating; (3) they can avoid the long waits experienced by N.H.S. patients; (4) they can often arrange for an operation to take place on a certain day of the week and at a certain time, thus minimizing the personal inconvenience involved.

An eminent British surgeon, who was the Regius Professor of Surgery at Oxford, explained why so many patients preferred private care:

They value their health and their lives. Also they put a value on their convenience and they don't want to wait. When they come to me they know I'm the top expert and I'm giving them the benefit of my knowledge and experience. I spend time with them in consultation. When they're to be operated on, I do the operation and I take care of them after surgery. I can arrange for them to be operated on quickly, maybe a few days or one or two weeks after the initial consultation. But on the National Health they have to take whatever junior person they get assigned; they don't know who's going to operate on them, and they realize the chances of getting me are slim. And they have to wait months or longer for the operation. So what they get when they pay is courtesy, time, my personal expert care, and the convenience of having the problem taken care of quickly. Don't you think that's worth paying for?[22]

The most important sentence in the above quotation is the first one. Is this merely a puffing statement of a man trying to enhance his market value? Or is it really true? This observation has been challenged, even by critics of the N.H.S. Enoch Powell, for example, doubts that the quality of care furnished outside the N.H.S. is superior to the quality of care furnished to Health Service patients.[23] And Professor Dennis Lees, an ardent critic of socialized medicine, has written that "there is no evidence at all that patients in private wards get better *clinical* care than those in public wards."[24]

But the views of Powell and Lees must surely be wrong. In London today there are consultants with international reputations who practice in teaching hospitals which are renowned throughout the world. A steady flow of patients from distant corners of the earth arrives there daily in search of private consultation and treatment. Most of the foreign patients come from the Middle East, North America and Europe.[25]

Are we to believe that Arab oil sheiks and wealthy Americans come to London for the standard of care meted out to the average British patient in an N.H.S. ward? Are we to believe that they would travel thousands of miles and spend thousands of dollars to be treated outside of London in worn-out, ill-equipped, 19th-century buildings, serviced by an inadequately-manned and undertrained staff, where most of the consultants have no merit award at all, where most of the hospital doctors are poorly-trained emigrants, to be operated upon by whomever the random luck-of-the-draw produces? The claim that private patients get the same clinical care received by the average N.H.S. patient is too ludicrous to be taken seriously.

There are, however, a number of complaints about private practice in N.H.S. hospitals that *do* seem to be legitimate. For instance, junior doctors and members of the hospitals' staff have complained that consultants often divert time, committed by their contracts to N.H.S. patients, to private patients; that they often allow N.H.S. patients to "jump the queue" in return for an initial private consultation; and that they do little to reduce their waiting lists in the hope that long waiting lists will persuade patients to "go private."[26] In addition, consultants have been accused of using ordinary N.H.S. beds to treat private patients. Complaints of this type have been so numerous that a parliamentary committee is currently investigating the abuses of private beds in government hospitals.[27]

Not surprisingly, what pay beds remain in N.H.S. hospitals are distributed very unequally. Of the approximately 4,000 pay beds, 25 percent are in London, and some regions of England, Scotland and Wales have less than 100.[28] The geographical distribution of pay beds by health regions is depicted in Table 8-2.[29]

Table 8-2

THE DISTRIBUTION OF PAY BEDS
(July, 1975)

Northern	169
Yorkshire	302
Trent	247
East Anglia	156
Thames, N.W.	461
Thames, N.E.	410
Thames, S.W.	247
Thames, S.E.	433
Wessex	191
Oxford	215
S. Western	205
West Midlands	394
Mersey	164
Northwestern	336
Post-graduate teaching hospitals	227

Source: John Roper, "Consultants Face Open Conflict with the State," *The* (London) *Times*, November 11, 1975.

Private Hospitals and Nursing Homes

Despite Britain's many economic troubles, a surprising growth industry is emerging: private hospitals. In 1978, there were 32,000 beds in private hospitals and nursing homes,[30] and many more are underway. In the spring of 1979, the Independent Hospital Group, a trade organization representing the private hospital industry in England, announced that 50 new private health care facilities are now in the planning or construction stage.[31]

One of the largest of the private companies is the Nuffield Nursing Homes Trust, which now operates 30 hospitals.[32] The market has also attracted American investors. American Medical International, for example, is now the largest investor in private medicine in the United Kingdom. In addition to its current holdings, the company is channeling $28 million into the construction of hospitals in Manchester, Harrow, and Windsor.[33]

Most private hospitals are fairly small. The number of beds, for instance, ranges up to about 150. There is also considerable variation in the number of services offered. Many are nursing homes without resident physicians.[34] But others are full-blown hospitals with international reputations. An example is the Wellington Hospital in London. The hospital is owned by an American firm, Humana, which manages two percent of all hospital beds in the U.S. About 60 to 70 percent of the hospital's patients come from the Middle East. Twenty percent of its patients are British, and another ten percent are from North America and Europe. Their operations include joint replacement, genitourinary surgery and, so far, 30 kidney transplants.[35]

The Wellington Hospital also illustrates another trend in British medicine. One entire floor has been taken over by 16 ophthalmic surgeons from Moorfields Hospital, an N.H.S. hospital where the private beds were recently closed.[36] Apparently the decline of private beds within the N.H.S. is being offset by a shift of beds and consultants to the private hospital sector.

Outside of London, private hospitals mainly treat the many non-urgent conditions for which N.H.S. patients may spend years awaiting treatment. The conditions include arthritis, gallstones, hernias and varicose veins.[37]

How important are the private hospitals? They are increasingly being seen as a safety valve for an over-worked, understaffed N.H.S. hospital sector. It is not uncommon, for example, for the N.H.S. to now place patients in private hospitals and private nursing homes for a contracted fee. Usually these are patients who need long-term or terminal care. In 1978, for example, the N.H.S. "rented" 3,133 beds (mostly for the elderly) in private hospitals and nursing homes.[38]

There are also examples of private clinics performing major surgery on N.H.S. patients. In 1978, two clinics operated by American Medical International accepted two N.H.S. patients for heart surgery. The case attracted considerable attention in the British press because N.H.S. doctors claimed that the two women patients were on a waiting list in an area where as many as 50 patients a year were dying for lack of heart surgery, and because American Medical International performed the operations free of charge — the Health

Service paid only for the heart valves and the transportation costs.[39]

As a profit-making firm, American Medical International may have looked upon these operations as more than altruistic gestures. The firm may need all of the good will it can muster if it wants to build more private hospitals. Authorization for private hospitals must be granted by the Health Services Board, which can refuse requests if it decides that a new private hospital will "jeopardize" the work of neighboring N.H.S. hospitals.[40] It is generally believed that the government will never allow the private sector to grow to the point where it is regarded as seriously undermining the N.H.S.[41]

This attitude is not uncommon, incidentally, in countries with national health insurance schemes. In Northern France recently, a group of radiologists wanted to purchase a CAT scanner for use in their private practice. But the French government refused to grant them an import license. The explanation given was that, until the state hospitals were able to afford scanners, they should not be available in private practice.[42]

Private Health Insurance

In 1966, a public opinion poll revealed that two-thirds of British citizens had never heard of private health insurance.[43] A poll taken today, however, would probably find much greater public awareness. As Figure 8-2 shows, the near doubling of subscribers in the last decade has made private health insurance another one of Britain's growth industries.

Figure 8-3 shows how most policies are being purchased these days — as a perquisite of employment. More and more British employers (including Kodak, Texaco, Ford and Laker Airways) have begun offering medical coverage as a fringe benefit to employees. Ninety-seven companies in *The* (London) *Times* list of the top 100 British corporations now provide some of their employees with private health insurance.[44]

In the early 1970s, private group health insurance was mainly offered to top company executives. In 1972, 17.3 percent of the executives in 580 companies surveyed were covered by health insurance policies. Five years later, the proportion of executives covered had grown to 38 percent. But the popularity of private health insurance is spreading to other workers as well — ten percent of the companies surveyed in 1978 offered free insurance to all of their employees.[45] Included among the blue collar holders of private health insurance are

Figure 8-2

SUBSCRIPTION INCOME
AND BENEFITS PAID
FOR PRIVATE MEDICAL
SCHEMES

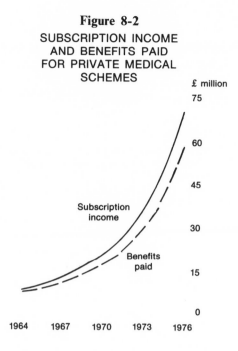

Source: UK Private Medical Care, Provident Schemes Statistics, 1974, Department
of Health and Social Security.

10,000 London taxi drivers and 45,000 members of the Electrical and
Plumbing Trades Union — the first major union to make private
health insurance an issue in collective bargaining.[46]

Part of the reason for the growth of private insurance as a fringe
benefit has been government-imposed wage and salary controls.
Fringe benefits were generally exempt from controls. So instead of
increasing a worker's salary by a certain number of dollars, the company could spend those same dollars on insurance premiums. But an
equally important reason often given is the "chaotic" state of the
N.H.S.

Figure 8-3
INSURANCE FOR PRIVATE MEDICAL CARE

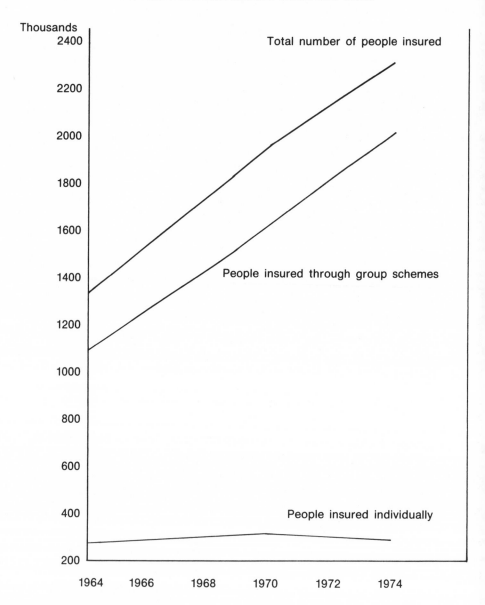

Footnotes

1. "Higher Still and Higher," *The Economist,* October 14, 1978, p. 107.
2. "Paying For Not Waiting," *The Economist,* July 29, 1978, p. 20.
3. Stuart Butler, "Thirty Years of National Health Care: A Review of the British Experience," (Washington, D.C.: Heritage Foundation, 1978), p. 19.
4. "Paying For Not Waiting," p. 20.
5. Richard Trubo, "Sources of Treatment," *The New York Times,* March 27, 1979.
6. "Private-School Boom," *Newsweek,* August 13, 1979, p. 83.
7. D. Mechanic, "Private Practice Among General Practitioners in the English National Health Service," *Medical Care,* July/August, 1970, pp. 324-332.
8. Ruth Levitt, *The Reorganized National Health Service* (London: Croom Helm, Ltd., 1976), p. 206.
9. Economic Models, Ltd., *The British Health Care System* (Chicago: American Medical Association, 1976), p. 147.
10. Ann Cartwright, *Patients and Their Doctors* (London: Routledge and Kegan Paul, 1967), p. 13.
11. Economic Models, Ltd., *The British Health Care System,* p. 147.
12. Cartwright, *Patients and Their Doctors,* p. 14.
13. "Receptionists Write Prescriptions," *The* (London) *Times,* January 28, 1977.
14. See Cartwright, *Patients and Their Doctors,* Ch. II.
15. A Cartwright and R. Marshall, "General Practice in 1963," *Medical Care,* 1965.
16. "N.H.S. in Crisis: Pay Beds Being Removed From Public Hospitals," *The* (London) *Times,* August 11, 1978.
17. Harry Swartz, "The Infirmity of British Medicine," in Emmett Tyrrell, ed., *The Future That Doesn't Work: Social Democracy's Failures in Britain* (New York: Doubleday, 1977), p. 37.
18. Butler, "Thirty Years of National Health Care," pp. 16-17.
19. See Puggy D. Nuttall, "The British National Health Service," *Nursing Outlook,* Vol 25, No. 2, February, 1977, p. 98.
20. Economic Models, Ltd., *The British Health Care System,* p. 149.
21. *Ibid,* p. 146.
22. Swartz, "The Infirmity of British Medicine," pp. 35-6.
23. Enoch Powell, *Medicine and Politics: 1975 and After* (New York: Pitman, 1976), p. 42.
24. Dennis Lees, "Economics and Non-economics of Health Services," *Three Banks Review,* 110, June, 1976, p. 18.
25. "N.H.S. in Crisis."
26. Economic Models, Ltd., *The British Health Care System,* p. 151.
27. *Ibid,* p. 122, n. 53.
28. Levitt, *The Reorganized National Health Service,* p. 207.
29. Statistics for years prior to 1974 are listed by Regional Hospital Boards (R.H.B.s); after 1974, the regions used are those of the Regional Health Authorities (R.H.A.s).
30. Economic Models, Ltd., *The British Health Care System,* p. 149.
31. Trubo, "Sources of Treatment."
32. "N.H.S. in Crisis."
33. Trubo, "Sources of Treatment."
34. "Private Care For the Elderly 'Important to N.H.S.'," *The* (London) *Times,* February 10, 1978.
35. "N.H.S. in Crisis."
36. *Ibid.*
37. *Ibid.*
38. "Private Care For the Elderly."
39. "An Affair of the Heart," *The Economist,* August 12, 1978, pp. 16-17.

40. *Ibid.*
41. Economic Models, Ltd., *The British Health Care System*, p. 152.
42. Anthony Lejeune, "Out the Window," *Private Practice*, May 1978, p. 42.
43. Stuart Butler and Eamonn Butler, *The British National Health Service in Theory and Practice: A Critical Analysis of Socialized Medicine* (Washington, D.C.: The Heritage Foundation, 1976), p. 47.
44. Trubo, "Sources of Treatment."
45. "Free Medicine Now a Perk," *The* (London) *Times*, March 6, 1978.
46. Jonathan Spivak, "Private Health Care in Britain," *Wall Street Journal*, August 21, 1979.

Chapter 9
Inequalities in the National Health Service

From the beginning, the concept of "equality" was central to the founders of the National Health Service. To Aneurin Bevan, the goal of equality was not merely a practical one to be traded off against other desirable ends. Bevan's argument was fundamentally a moral one: "Everyone should be treated alike in the mother of medical care."[1]

Precisely what does this statement mean? An uncharitable interpretation would be to take the statement literally. By definition, the "best" doctors are limited in number. Not everyone can have access to them. The only way to achieve genuine equality in physician care is to eliminate the best. For while the best are limited in number, the mediocre are more numerous; the inferior more numerous still.

Genuine equality could be achieved only by lowering the standard of care in ways that would certainly be inhumane. It could be achieved by mandating that, unless all kidney patients can have optimal treatment, none shall have it; unless all candidates for a brain scan can have one, none shall have one; unless all candidates for heart surgery can have the operation, none shall be operated upon. But even this path is illusory. For in deciding to treat some medical conditions and not others, we would necessarily be discriminating. We would necessarily be implying that the medical needs of some are more important than the medical needs of others — which is hardly the way to treat everyone alike.

Bevan, of course, did not envision a general lowering of the standards of medical care, nor did the other founding fathers of the N.H.S. The Beveridge Report proposed "a health service providing full preventive and curative treatment of every kind for every citizen without exceptions."[2] The British Medical Journal predicted that the N.H.S. was to be "a 100 per cent service for 100 per cent of the population."[3]

The most charitable thing that can be said about the proponents of socialized medicine is that their vision was terribly muddled and confused. One thing is quite clear, however: whatever inequalities that were permitted to exist were not to be based on age, sex, occupation, geographical location, or — most important of all — income and social class. As Bevan put it, "the essence of a satisfactory health service is that rich and poor are treated alike, that poverty is not a disability and wealth is not advantaged."[4]

How does the N.H.S. measure up in terms of these objectives? Very poorly. It is now an open question in Britain — among the N.H.S. critics and defenders alike — whether the Health Service has in any way produced more equality in the consumption of medical care than would otherwise have existed. This is especially true with respect to the most hated of all distinctions — social class. A very common view today is represented by the comments of Dr. Tony Smith, a health services correspondent for *The* (London) *Times*. In 1978, Smith wrote that "the differences between the social classes have widened rather than narrowed in the 30 years of the N.H.S."[5] In each of the previous chapters we have presented evidence of inequality — and in some cases extreme inequality — in the provision of various types of medical services. In this chapter, we shall briefly summarize that evidence and look at some additional studies that have recently been completed.

Inequality: Geography and Medical Need

One of the easiest types of inequality to measure is inequality in the geographical distribution of health services. This is because the government regularly collects information on the amount of spending by each health region. Table 9-1 summarizes the geographical distribution of per capita health expenditures for three types of health services: hospital services, community health services, and general practitioner services.

Spending statistics for each of these services were presented separately in previous chapters. The new insight provided by Table 9-1 is that, as a general rule, regions where per capita spending is high for one type of health service are the very same regions where per capita spending is high for other types of services. The converse holds true for regions where per capita spending is low. For example, for each dollar spent on hospital services for a resident of the N.W. Thames region, only 67.4 cents is spent on behalf of a resident of Trent; and for each dollar spent in N.W. Thames on community health and general practitioner services, only 80.3 cents is spent on a resident of Trent. Overall, for every health dollar spent on an in-

Table 9-1

CURRENT EXPENDITURE PER CAPITA, BY REGION

	Hospital Services £	% of mean	Community health and family practitioner service £	% of mean	Total[1] £	% of mean
Northern	56.19	90.98	28.42	100.39	100.13	95.47
Yorkshire	56.86	92.07	27.42	96.86	97.44	92.91
Trent	50.49	81.75	26.67	94.21	93.80	89.44
East Anglia	53.83	87.16	26.94	95.16	95.22	90.79
N.W. Thames	74.91	121.29	33.21	117.31	122.38	116.69
N.E. Thames	76.35	123.62	25.95	91.66	117.00	111.56
S.E. Thames	73.61	119.19	29.28	103.43	118.17	112.67
S.W. Thames	67.00	108.48	28.67	101.27	112.73	107.48
Wessex	52.44	84.91	28.15	99.43	94.00	89.63
Oxford	53.18	86.11	28.23	99.72	96.09	91.62
South Western	57.87	93.70	30.50	107.74	103.33	98.52
West Midlands	52.65	85.25	26.96	95.23	91.52	87.26
Mersey	62.16	100.65	27.92	98.62	107.16	102.17
North Western	57.63	93.31	28.88	102.01	100.46	95.79

1. Includes "headquarters administration," "other services" and capital expenditure not shown separately.

Source: *Royal Commission on the National Health Service Report* (Merrison Report) (London: Her Majesty's Stationery Office, 1979), Table 3.1, p. 15.

dividual in the N.W. Thames region, only 76.7 cents is spent on a resident of Trent.

These numbers probably understate the true inequality in the geographical distribution of health services. As we saw in chapter 6, inequalities in the distribution of spending are far greater *within* the health regions than *among* the health regions. Table 6-8 illustrated how wide these inequalities are in the hospital sector. On the basis of the pattern depicted in Table 9-1, as well as other evidence, there is every reason to believe that the inequalities are just as great for local authority and general practitioner services.

While Table 9-1 tells a great deal about spending, it tells us nothing about medical *need*. Is it possible that those regions with the largest per capita spending are regions with the greatest medical need? The answer is *no*. Table 9-2 shows how health service spending correlates with some crude indicators of medical need.

A region with a high birth rate would presumably have a greater need for maternity services than a region with a low birth rate. Similarly, since the medical needs of the aged are typically much greater than the medical needs of the rest of the population, a region with

Table 9-2

CORRELATIONS BETWEEN HEALTH AND SOCIAL STATUS
INDICATORS AND HEALTH SERVICE PER CAPITA SPENDING

	Community health expenditure	Hospital revenue expenditure	Hospital capital expenditure
Birth rate	-0.6388	-0.5242	-0.0580
Death rate	0.2420	0.0324	-0.3318
% population over 65	0.3600	0.1227	-0.1268
Infant mortality rate	-0.4458	-0.3305	-0.2626
% of population managerial and professional	0.8307	0.7937	0.4700
% of population semi-skilled and unskilled manual	-0.7455	-0.7822	-0.2314

Source: J. Noyce, A. A. Snaith and A. J. Trickey, "Regional Variations in the Allocation of Financial Resources to the Community Health Services," *The Lancet*, March 30, 1974, Table III, p. 556.

a higher proportion of elderly citizens would presumably have a much greater need for health services than a region with a low proportion. Infant mortality rates and population mortality rates are also thought to be indicators of overall health needs. In general, high mortality rates are indicative of a low standard of health among the population.

Table 9-2 can be interpreted in the following way: a positive number indicates a positive correlation between a type of spending and an indicator of health need. In other words, more need, more spending. A negative number indicates a negative correlation: more need, less spending. The size of these numbers (in absolute terms) is also important. The larger the number, the greater the degree of correlation. In addition, larger numbers are numbers about which we can be more confident. For example, if the number is .7800, we can be very confident that the relationship *really* is positive and not the result of a statistical fluke. Similarly, if the number is -.7800, we can be very confident that the relationship *really* is negative. Conversely, we can have little confidence about numbers in the + or - .2 range.[6]

What Table 9-2 shows is that there is no systematic, positive relationship between spending and need, and in some cases there is a perverse (negative) relationship. Higher births are associated with *lower* per capita spending of all three kinds. There is no significant relationship between population mortality rates and spending. And there is a *negative* (but not highly significant) relationship between infant mortality and all three kinds of spending.

Inequality: The Role of Social Class

The most surprising result in Table 9-2, however, is the strong positive association between health service spending and social class. There is a highly significant positive relationship between health service spending and the percentage of the population working in managerial and professional occupations. Conversely, there is a highly significant negative relationship between health service spending and the percentage of the population working in semi-skilled and unskilled jobs.

These results are probably not shocking to close observers of the N.H.S. Indeed, in Britain these results probably conform with what most people would have guessed. Nonetheless, they are at odds with the British government's own assessment of the role of the N.H.S. in British economic life. The Central Statistical Office (C.S.O.), for example, maintains that the N.H.S. plays a crucial role in redistributing income from high-income to low-income groups. In fact, the C.S.O. finds that health benefits improve the distribution of income more than housing subsidies, family allowances or educational expenditure.[7] The trouble with this finding is that it is based on statistical assumptions that no conscientious researcher can begin to accept.

More light has recently been cast on this subject by Julian Le-Grand, Professor of Economics at the University of Sussex.[8] Professor LeGrand recently obtained access to previously unavailable data, and used a novel methodology to arrive at the results shown in Table 9-3.

Table 9-3

THE DISTRIBUTION OF PUBLIC EXPENDITURE ON HEALTH CARE IN ENGLAND AND WALES, 1972

Socioeconomic group	% of total reporting either limiting long-standing illness or acute sickness	% of health care expenditure	Ratio of expenditure per person reporting ill to that for SEGs V and VI
	(1)	(2)	(3)
I and II: Professionals, employers and managers	13.9	16.8	1.41
III: Intermediate and junior non-manual	19.7	22.5	1.33
IV: Skilled manual and own account non-professional	34.5	33.4	1.13
V and VI: Semi- and unskilled manual	31.9	27.3	1.00

Source: Julian LeGrand, "The Distribution of Public Expenditure: The Case of Health Care," *Economica,* Vol. 45, No. 178, May, 1978.

Table 9-3 can be interpreted as follows: columns (1) and (2) show that individuals in the professional and managerial class comprise about 14 percent of the total of those reporting ill, yet receive almost 17 percent of the total amount spent by the N.H.S. in the form of health services. By contrast, semi-skilled and unskilled workers comprise about 32 percent of those reporting illness, yet receive little more than 27 percent of the total amount spent on health services.[9]

Column (3) shows another way of looking at these same results. This shows the ratio of expenditure per person in each social class to the expenditure per person in the lowest social class. It can be seen that individuals in the professional and managerial class benefit from about 40 percent more spending than do individuals in the lowest social class. Put another way, if an individual in the highest social class becomes ill, he can expect that about 40 percent more health-care dollars will be spent on his treatment than on an individual with the same illness in the lowest social class.

If anything, the results in Table 9-3 probably understate the true amount of socioeconomic inequality in the distribution of health-care benefits. For example, while LeGrand obtained data on how many G.P. visits were made by members of each social class, he made no allowance for differences in time spent with the physician. So he simply attributed the average cost of a G.P. visit to each visit that he had recorded. Similarly, LeGrand assumed that the cost of out-patient consultations and in-patient stays did not vary across social classes.

The assumptions, as LeGrand admits,[10] bias his results in the direction of more equality. We saw in Chapter 5 that a number of studies have found that members of the highest social class spend from 40 to 50 percent more time with their G.P.s than members of the lowest social class. It seems likely that similar differentials exist for out-patient consultations.

In addition, out-patient and in-patient hospital costs are hardly uniform across the social classes. The cost per patient for out-patient and in-patient hospital care, for example, is from 40 to 50 percent greater in a London teaching hospital than in a non-teaching hospital. The costs are 20 to 30 percent greater in provincial teaching hospitals than in non-teaching hospitals.[11] It seems highly probable that access to these teaching hospitals is positively related to the patients' social class.

A reasonable guess, then, would be that members of the highest social class receive anywhere from one-and-one-half to two times as many health care dollars as do members of the lowest social class for any given illness.

Note that our discussion so far has been couched entirely in terms of the amount of money that is spent. We have said nothing about quality. Yet, despite the absence of money prices in the N.H.S., quality certainly has a market value. Indeed, the increasing recognition of "clear social class gradients in the use of health facilities"[12] by academic researchers, and the persistent references to the "Inverse Care Law" in the British press, probably reflect judgments about the quality of care received far more than they reflect judgments about the number of dollars spent.

British health economist Anthony Culyer recently reflected on much of the evidence we have been discussing, and asked a simple question:

> Why is this so? In Britain, health care treatment is free of money charges, so why should those who are, on the whole, poorer appear to demand less than one would predict simply on the basis of incidence of disease?[13]

In Chapter 5, we considered some possible answers to this question as it pertained to the general practitioner sector of the N.H.S. Professor LeGrand believes that many of these same answers are applicable to other sectors of the N.H.S. as well.[14] In general, schemes of non-price rationing seem to discriminate against low-income individuals. The barriers of non-price rationing appear to be as, or more, formidable than price.

A more basic question, though, is: why does the British government not make a more concerted effort to eliminate obvious inequalities in health care services? Why does the government not make access to health care easier for low-income individuals? Why does it not devote more N.H.S. resources to those sectors of the N.H.S. where the poor would derive the greatest benefit?

There has certainly been no lack of official pronouncements of intent. Recently, former Minister of Health David Owen declared that "the ultimate abolition of the present inequalities in health provision and care is ... the central task for the National Health Service over the next five years."[15] But, as we have seen, according to Bevan, that was supposed to have been the central task all along!

Almost a decade ago, Michael Cooper and Anthony Culyer argued that

> The major indictment of the National Health Service's first 20 years is the lack of any real efforts to determine the problems and to evolve and implement techniques for achieving in a national way the objective of equality.[16]

Their observation that no "real efforts" have been made to achieve the objective of equality is probably as valid today as it was ten years ago. To see why no efforts have been made, we need to take a close look at the politics of medicine.

Footnotes

1. Quoted in Economic Models, Ltd., *The British Health Care System* (Chicago: American Medical Association, 1976), p. 33.
2. Quoted in Harry Swartz, "The Infirmity of British Medicine," in Emmett Tyrrell, Jr., ed., *The Future That Doesn't Work: Social Democracy's Failures in Britain* (New York: Doubleday, 1977), p. 24.
3. *British Medical Journal,* December 12, 1942, p. 700.
4. Aneurin Bevan, *In Place of Fear* (London: Heinemann, 1952), p. 76.
5. Dr. Tony Smith, "Verdict on N.H.S.: Could Do Better," *The* (London) *Times,* July 5, 1978.
6. In statistical terminology, coefficients .78 are significant at 0.1% level; 0.6614 at 1% level, and 0.5325 at 5% level.
7. Central Statistical Office, "Effects of Taxes and Benefits on Household Income 1975," *Economic Trends* (London: Her Majesty's Stationery Office, 1976), particularly pp. 105 and 111.
8. Julian LeGrand, "The Distribution of Public Expenditure: The Case of Health Care, *Economica,* Vol. 45, No. 178, May, 1978.
9. The statistics have also been standardized for age and sex differences among the social classes. Age-sex standardized data give approximately the same results as those shown in Table 9-3. See, LeGrand, "The Distribution of Public Expenditure," Table 2, p. 131.
10. *Ibid,* pp. 132-3.
11. Economic Models, Ltd., *The British Health Care System,* p. 56.
12. Kenneth Lee, "Public Expenditure, Planning and Local Democracy," in Keith Barnard and Kenneth Lee, eds., *Conflicts in the National Health Service* (London: Croom Helm, 1977), p. 223.
13. Anthony Culyer, *Need and the National Health Service* (Towata, New Jersey: Rowman and Littlefield, 1976) p. 22.
14. LeGrand, "The Distribution of Public Expenditure," pp. 136-8.
15. David Owen, *In Sickness and In Health* (London: Quartet, 1976), p. 60.
16. Michael Cooper and Anthony Culyer, "An Economic Assessment of Some Aspects of the Operation of the National Health Service," in British Medical Association, *Health Services Financing* (London: British Medical Association, 1970), p. 207.

Chapter 10
The Politics of Medicine

Many of the characteristics of the British system of socialized medicine can be explained on the basis of economic principles alone. In Chapter 4, we identified a number of the most important of these principles. In Chapters 5 through 8 we showed how these principles could be used to analyze the various sectors of the N.H.S. In general, the absence of money prices in the market for health care leads to long waiting lines, reduced quality and substantial inefficiencies in the delivery of health care.

Other characteristics of the N.H.S., however, cannot be explained simply by reference to economic principles. These are characteristics which arise as a result of *political choices*. They include: (1) the decision about how much to spend on health services; (2) the decision to permit widespread inequalities in the consumption of health care; (3) the decision to sacrifice "curing" services to "caring" services; (4) the decision to sacrifice capital expenditure to current expenditure; (5) the decision to leave most administrative decisions within the N.H.S. to producer interest groups; and (6) the decision to retain the system of socialized medical care rather than switch to some clear alternatives.

A curious paradox pervades most discussions of the N.H.S. With increasing frequency, academic researchers today are accepting the fact that economic principles *do* apply to the market for health care. Yet, almost without exception, commentaries on the N.H.S. imply that there are no political principles governing the health care policies of the British government.

An example to illustrate this paradox may help. In the Middle Ages, it was common to speak of the "just price" of goods and services sold in the marketplace. Prices above or below this price were considered "unjust." This way of looking at prices was, naturally, closely connected with an evaluation of the character of market participants — usually the sellers of goods and services. A seller who charged a price higher than the "just price" was a seller who had a character defect — he had succumbed to temptation and committed the sin of avarice or greed.

Today, this view of the marketplace is universally rejected as hogwash. We now know that market prices have almost nothing to do with the character of the participants in the market. In general, sellers have very little choice about what prices they charge, just as consumers have very little choice about what prices they pay. Prices in the marketplace are understood to be the outcome of fundamental market forces — forces over which individual buyers and sellers have very little control.

The science of economics, then, has come a long way over the last several centuries. No modern economist would try to explain a market price by reference to the characters or personalities of producers and sellers. Explanation in economics today is totally divorced from psychology and ethics. Explanation in economics is always explanation by reference to fundamental economic *principles*.

In the science of politics, however, things are very different. Political science today is barely beginning to emerge from the stage it occupied in the Middle Ages. Hence, it is still quite common to speak of "just laws" in the same way in which people used to speak of "just prices." Presumably, "just laws" are laws passed by "just" politicians; whereas "unjust" laws are the product of politicians who suffer from character defects.

The consequence of this very primitive view of politics is the tendency to explain important pieces of legislation by reference to the character, intelligence and personality of politicians. It is evident in the widespread view that if only politicians were more intelligent, better educated or more moral, we would have very different political policies. Note that this viewpoint implicitly assumes that politicians have an enormous amount of choice, and that they are not driven to do what they do by fundamental political forces.

In calling this viewpoint "primitive," I am not asserting that fundamental notions of "right" and "wrong" are not important in politics. They are important. But they are important in the same way in which they are important in the economic marketplace. Fundamental notions of right and wrong influence which products will be purchased by consumers. Similarly, they influence which politicians and which political policies will be acceptable to voters.

But there is no reason to suppose that the politician who trades political policies for votes has any more freedom of choice than the entrepreneur who trades goods and services for money. To the contrary; recent developments in the theory of politics suggest that the laws which are produced in the political marketplace, just like the prices which are produced in the economic marketplace, are determined by fundamental forces — forces over which the individual politician has little, if any, control.

Public Choice Theory

"Public Choice" is the name given to a relatively new discipline which, in many ways, attempts to integrate economics and political science.[1] Its chief goal is to attempt to explain political phenomena by reference to fundamental principles, in much the same way that economists explain purely economic phenomena. The name, however, is potentially misleading. The new discipline could just as easily be called "modern political science."

One of the most fascinating developments in this discipline is the discovery that a number of economic principles, if used with care, can help explain much of what happens in politics. Take the concept of competition. Just as producers of goods and services compete for consumer dollars, so politicians, in a democracy, compete for votes. Moreover, the process of competition leads to certain well-defined results.

In the economic marketplace, competition inevitably forces producers to choose the lowest-cost method of production. Producers who fail to discover or to implement the lowest-cost method of production suffer financial losses. They either go out of business or mend their ways. The ultimate outcome then — efficient production — is independent of any particular producer's wishes or desires.

In a similar way, political competition inexorably leads political candidates to adopt a specific political position. It's called the *winning platform*. The idea of a winning platform is a fairly simple one. It is a set of political policies (a platform) that can defeat any other set of policies in an election. A politician who wants to be elected, or who wants to remain in office, has every incentive to endorse the winning platform. If he adopts some other platform, he becomes vulnerable. For if an opposing politician adopts the winning platform and he does not, the opponent will win the election.

Of course in the real world, things are rarely that simple. Many factors influence voters other than substantive political issues — a candidate's religion, general appearance, speaking ability, party affiliation, etc. Moreover, even when voters are influenced by real political issues, politicians often don't know what the winning platform really is. Often they must guess at its location. Nonetheless, the theory holds that, other things being equal, a candidate always improves his chances of winning by endorsing the winning platform. Hence, all candidates have an incentive to try to discover what the winning platform is and to endorse it. Those candidates who refuse to do this are unlikely to survive the political competition.

This line of reasoning leads to a remarkable conclusion: in democratic political systems, with two major political parties, there is always a tendency for both parties to adopt the same political policies. They do so not because the party leaders think alike or share the same ideological preferences, but because their top priority is to win elections and hold political office.

Two corollaries follow from this conclusion. The first is that it is absurd to complain about the fact that "major candidates all sound alike," or that "it doesn't seem to make any difference who wins." These complaints are merely evidence that political competition is working precisely as the theory predicts it will work. Indeed, as political candidates get more accurate information because of better polling techniques and the use of the computer, the more similar they will become. The theory predicts that, in a world of perfect information, the policies of the two major parties would be identical.

The second corollary is more relevant for our purposes. Put in its extreme form, the corollary asserts that "politicians don't matter." Over the long haul, if we want to explain why we have the political policies we have, it is futile to investigate the motives, personalities and characters of those politicans who actually held office. Instead we must focus on those factors which determine the nature of the winning platform.

This corollary is crucially important to an understanding of the British system of socialized medicine. A great many British health economists, including Anthony Culyer and Michael Cooper, are quick to concede that the N.H.S. has many defects. But these defects, in their view, are not the defects of socialism; they merely represent a failure of political will, or the fact that the wrong politicians were in office. The ultimate goal, it is held, is to retain the system of socialized medicine and make it work better.

By contrast, I shall argue in the remainder of this chapter that the defects of the political policies which govern the N.H.S. are *natural and inevitable consequences* of placing the market for health under the control of politicians. It is not the case that British health care policy just happened to be as it is but could have been different.

Alone among British commentators, Enoch Powell seems to have appreciated this fact. Powell writes that "whatever is entrusted to politicians becomes political even if it is not political anyhow,"[2] and goes on to say that

> The phenomena of Medicine and Politics ... result automatically and necessarily from the nationalization of medical care and its provision gratis at the point of consumption ... [T]hese phenomena are implicit in such an organization and are not the accidental or incidental results of blemishes which can be 'reformed' away while leaving the system as such intact.[3]

The Total Amount of Spending on Health Services

One of the arguments used to justify socialized medicine is that, left to their own devices, individuals will not spend as much as they *ought* to spend on health care. In Chapter 2, we saw that this was one of the major reasons why many middle- and upper-middle-class citizens supported national health insurance for the working-class. It was also a major reason for the support for the N.H.S. in 1948.[4] A great many people expected that, under socialized medical care, more total dollars would be spent on health care than would otherwise have been the case.

In fact, it is not clear that socialized medicine in Britain has increased the overall amount of spending on health care. It may have even led to the *opposite* result. This is the contention of Dennis Lees, Professor of Economics at the University of Nottingham. Lees has argued for years that the N.H.S. has led to less spending than would otherwise have occurred. As recently as 1976, for example, he wrote that "the British people, left free to do so, would almost certainly have chosen to spend more on health services themselves than governments have chosen to spend on their behalf."[5]

Is Lees correct? It is difficult to prove the contention conclusively, but there is plenty of evidence to support the indictment. As we saw in Chapter 3, total N.H.S. spending in 1965 was the same percentage (about 4.2 percent) of gross national product as it was fifteen years earlier in 1950. This is an amazing result in the light of what we know about the private demand for health care. International studies show a strong and significant positive relationship between a country's GNP and the percent of GNP spent on health care.[6] In general, the wealthier the country, the greater the percent of its income that it spends on medical care. Not only does this relationship hold across countries at a point in time, but it also holds *within* countries over time. The relationship, for example, has been shown to exist over time in the United States and Japan — two countries with large private medical care sectors.[7]

In addition to the statistical evidence, public choice theory suggests that under socialized medical systems there is a tendency to spend less on health care than people, on the average, would have spent in the private marketplace. To see why this is true, let us first imagine a situation in which a politician is trying to win the vote of a single voter. To keep the example simple, let us suppose the politician has access to $10 to spend on the voter's behalf. The politician can spend this money on health services, social security benefits, family allowances or dozens of other programs. If the goal is to get elected or re-elected, though, how should the politician best spend it?

The answer is fairly simple. To maximize his chance of winning the voter's vote, the politician should spend the $10 precisely as the voter wants it spent. So if the voter's choice is $5 in the form of medical care, $3 in the form of a retirement pension, and $2 in the form of a rent subsidy, that should also be the choice of the vote-maximizing politician. If the politician does not choose to spend the $10 in this way, he risks losing this voter's vote to a clever opponent.

Now it might seem that if the voter wants $5 spent on medical care, we can conclude that he would have spent the $5 on medical care himself *if* he were spending $10 of his own money. But this is not quite true. State-provided medical care has one feature that is generally missing from private medical markets and from other government spending programs as well — non-price rationing. Non-price rationing, as we have seen, imposes heavy costs on patients (such as the cost of waiting and other inconveniences), leads to deterioration in the quality of service rendered, and creates many other forms of waste and inefficiency.

This means that, other things being equal, $5 of spending through the N.H.S. will be a lot less valuable to the average voter than $5 of spending in a private market for medical care. It also means that, under socialized medicine, spending for health care will be less attractive to voters relative to spending programs which do not involve non-price rationing.

Public choice theory, then, predicts that the average voter will desire less spending on health care, relative to other goods and services, when health care is rationed by non-market devices. Moreover, the greater the rationing problems, the less attractive health care spending will be. So we would expect even less spending on health care in a completely "free" service like the N.H.S. than we would in a health service that tacked on more user fees, as many other countries do.

Of course in the real world, politicians rarely have the opportunity to tailor their spending to the specific desires of specific voters. Generally the politician must allocate spending among programs that affect thousands of voters at the same time. New spending for a hospital, for example, provides benefits for every one in the surrounding community. No matter what level of spending is chosen, some voters will have preferred more spending, while others will have preferred less. In general, the vote-maximizing level of spending will be the level of spending preferred by the average voter.

Inequalities in the National Health Service

Like the decision about how much to spend on health services, the decision about *where* to spend health dollars is also an inherently political decision. A major argument in favor of the N.H.S. was that the system of private medical care led to geographical inequalities in levels of provision. Yet, as we have seen, those inequalities continue to persist, and many critics argue that levels of provision across living areas of Britain today are just as unequal as they would have been in the absence of the N.H.S.

In theory, creating regional equality is a relatively simple task. All the British government has to do is spend more in areas that are relatively deprived and spend less in areas that are relatively well-endowed. But the British government has not done this. Why? Public choice theory supplies a possible answer.

Policy-makers must make two choices about spending in a particular area or region. First, they must decide how many total dollars are to be spent in the area. Second, they must decide how to allocate those dollars among alternative programs. In a democracy, there is no particular reason *why* per capita spending will be the same in all areas.

Per capita spending may differ across voting districts for numerous reasons. Voter turnout may be higher in some districts than in others. This means that some districts may be willing to "pay" more (in terms of votes) in return for political largesse. The voters in some districts may be more aware of, and more sensitive to, any changes in per capita spending than voters in other districts.

Given that a certain amount of money is going to be spent in a certain area or region, competition for votes dictates that the money be allocated in accordance with the preference of the voters in that area or region. To return to the hypothetical example of the previous section, suppose that, say, $10 is going to be spent in the city of Merseyside. If a majority of residents want $2 spent on health services and $8 spent on other programs, political competition will tend to produce that result. Yet if the residents of some other city want $8 spent on health services and $2 spent on other programs, political competition will also tend to produce that result.

Prior to the N.H.S., geographical inequalities reflected community preferences. In general, the citizens of wealthier and more densely populated areas chose to spend a larger fraction of their income on medical care than did the citizens of less wealthy and more sparsely populated areas. There is no reason to suppose that these preferences were radically altered after the introduction of the N.H.S. Hence, there is no reason to suppose that in allocating public spending, vote-maximizing politicians are doing anything other than responding to voter preferences.

Spending Priorities: "Caring" Versus "Curing"

One of the most remarkable features of the N.H.S. is the emphasis given to what we have described as "caring" rather than "curing" aspects of medical care. This feature of the N.H.S. marks a radical difference between British and American health care.

Numerous examples of the "caring" versus "curing" distinction were given in Chapter 6. There we noted that the N.H.S. finances 20.1 million non-emergency ambulance rides each year, but refuses to staff its ambulances with paramedics or emergency medical technicians. The N.H.S. spends almost as much on "free" eyesight tests each year as it spends on dialysis machines, even though thousands of British citizens die each year for lack of dialysis. The N.H.S. finances eight million house calls by home nurses and health visitors each year, but refuses to buy more than a handful of life-saving CAT scanners.

There can be no doubt that these choices reflect the pressures of the political process. They are the result of conscious political decisions. And the current trend is toward even more "caring" and less "curing." American economist Mary-Ann Rozbicki recently asked a number of British health planners the following question: "If you suddenly enjoyed a sharp increase in available resources, how would you allocate it?" The response was invariably the same. They would put the additional resources into services for the aged, the chronically ill and the mentally handicapped.[8]

Commenting on this response, Rozbicki writes:

It is difficult for an American observer to comprehend that view. He has been impressed by the support services already afforded the non-acute patient (and the well consumer) — the doctor, nurse, and social worker attendance at homes, clinics and hospitals for the purpose of improving the comfort and well-being of the recipients involved. He has also been impressed (and sometimes shocked) by the relative lack of capability to diagnose, cure, and/or treat life-threatening conditions. The U.S. patient, while having forgone the home ministrations of the family doctor and learned to endure the antiseptic quality of the hospital, also confidently expects immediate delivery of all that medical science has to offer if life or health is under immediate threat.[9]

What political pressures lead decision makers to prefer the "caring" functions of medical care over the "curing" functions? Rozbicki believes it is a matter of numbers — *numbers of votes*. Money spent on "caring" services is spread out over far more people than money spent on "curing" services. Rozbicki writes:

In weighing the choice between a more comfortable life for the millions of aged or early detection and treatment of the far fewer victims of dread diseases, [the British health authorities] have favored the former. In choosing between a fully equipped hospital therapy and rehabilitation center or nuclear medicine technology, they have favored the former. *The sheer numbers involved on each side of the equation would tend to dictate these choices by government officials in a democratic society.*[10]

Rozbicki's insight may be correct. But it cannot be a complete explanation. It is true that the number of potential beneficiaries of home visiting far exceeds the number of potential beneficiaries of an equivalent amount of spending on radiation therapy. But all British citizens are potentially ill. Thus all British citizens have an interest in the spending priorities of the N.H.S. A complete explanation for these priorities requires us to explain why the average citizen would approve of them.

Like the citizens of other countries, most British citizens know very little about the technology of medical care. This ignorance, moreover, is quite "rational." Information is costly. The rational person has an incentive to expand his knowledge about any subject *only* up to the point where the cost of an additional bit of information is equal to its benefit. This is the economic explanation for the commonly-observed fact that the average person does not acquire expert knowledge in the field of medical science.

In Britain, however, the average citizen has much less of an incentive to become knowledgeable about medicine than his counterpart in the United States. The reason is that, in Britain, medical care is socialized. In the U.S., if a person becomes more knowledgeable about medical matters, this knowledge can often yield a direct personal benefit. Precisely because the medical market in the U.S. is largely private, a more informed person becomes a more intelligent consumer — he is in a better position to know whether or not to purchase any particular medical service.

But within the confines of the N.H.S., medical services are not "purchased." Suppose a British citizen invests his time and money to learn more about medical matters and discovers, lo and behold, that the N.H.S. is not offering the kinds of services it ought to offer. Of what possible value is this knowledge? It is of virtually no personal value unless the citizen can inform millions of other voters, persuade them to "throw the rascals out," and achieve a change of policy. But such a campaign would be enormously expensive, and would undoubtedly promise to cost the citizen far more than any potential personal benefit he could expect to derive from it.

Socialized medicine affects the level of knowledge that patients have in yet another way. In a free market for medical care, suppliers of medical services have an incentive to inform potential customers about new developments in medicine. Such information increases the demand for new services and, thus, promises to enhance the income of those who supply them. In the N.H.S., however, the suppliers of medical care have no such incentives. Doctors, nurses and hospital administrators increase their income chiefly by persuading the government to pay them more. They increase their comfort, leisure time, and other forms of satisfaction by encouraging patients not to demand more, but to demand *less*.

Economic theory, then, would predict that in a socialized medical scheme, people will acquire less knowledge about medical care than they would have acquired in a private system of medical care. The evidence confirms this prediction. Numerous commentators have observed that British patients know far less about medical care than American patients. Rozbicki, for example, writes that "the British populace appears much less sophisticated in its medical demands" than the American populace.[11]

The general ignorance about medical science which prevails among British voters has a profound impact on N.H.S. policies. Other things being equal, people will always place a higher value on those services with which they are more familiar than on those goods and services with which they are less familiar. Other things being equal, they will place a higher value on benefits about which they are certain than on benefits about which they are uncertain. The known is preferred to the unknown. Certainty is preferred to uncertainty. The average British voter is familiar with, and fairly certain about, the personal value of the non-acute services provided by the N.H.S. He is probably unfamiliar with, and uncertain about, the personal value of acute services which could be provided to many more patients. This is one of the reasons why the average British voter will tend to approve of the N.H.S. spending priorities.

There is also another reason why voters will tend to prefer "caring" to "curing" services in health care. This reason stems from a characteristic of *non-price rationing*. All of the services of the N.H.S. require rationing. But in some sectors, the rationing problems are far greater than in others. This is because, for some types of medical services, quality can be sacrificed to quantity. We have seen that, in comparison with American doctors, British G.P.s have greatly reduced the time spent with each patient and the quality of service rendered. Nonetheless, this type of adjustment allows the typical patient to actually visit his G.P. within two or three days of making an appointment. The quality of treatment may have deteriorated, but patients are at least certain that they will receive *some* treatment. Presumably, this is the type of adjustment patients prefer given the overall rationing problem.

These kinds of adjustments, however, cannot be made with most acute services. A CAT scan is a CAT scan. An organ transplant is an organ transplant. Renal dialysis is renal dialysis. In general, there is no feasible way to sacrifice quality for quantity in these areas. Patients seeking these services must simply live with uncertainty. They will either receive full treatment or no treatment. Very few patient-pleasing adjustments can be made to ease the burdens of non-price rationing.

These characteristics of health care rationing have an important effect on the preferences of potential patients — even patients who are very knowledgeable about medicine. The existence of non-price rationing tends to make all health care services less valuable to potential patients than those services would be in the free market. But because non-acute services can be adjusted to increase the certainty of some treatment, whereas acute services generally cannot be so adjusted, the former will tend to become more valuable *relative to* the latter. Thus, to a certain extent, the priority given to non-acute treatment is a perfectly rational phenomenon for citizens living under a socialized medical scheme.

Spending Priorities: Current Expenditure Versus Capital Expenditure

Closely related to the distinction between the "caring" and "curing" aspects of British medical care is the distinction between current expenditure and capital expenditure. As we saw in Chapter 6, the N.H.S. has favored the former over the latter. Despite the fact that the N.H.S. inherited a deteriorating capital stock, only one new hospital was built in the first 15 years of operation. Even today, over 50 percent of the hospital beds are in buildings built in the nineteenth century. Moreover, there are fewer hospital beds today than there were when the N.H.S. was founded.

Capital expenditure, as we have seen, creates a flow of benefits which extend many years into the future. Current expenditure, by definition, creates benefits which are realized in the current period. The distinction between the two types of expenditure, then, is largely a distinction between benefits later and benefits now. The political preference of the British is quite clear. They prefer benefits now. Can public choice theory help us explain this preference? Indeed it can. To see how, we first need to consider how decisions about capital spending are made in the free market.

Very few of us probably know how our consumption of, say, coffee varies over the seasons of the year. Most of us simply buy coffee when we want it and, except for the influence of general inflation or an occasional coffee tree blight in Brazil, we pay about the same price regardless of the month of the year. But this fact is in itself rather amazing. At the end of each year's coffee harvest, why don't we see the entire supply of coffee dumped on the market and sold at very low prices? That is, why isn't coffee abundant and low-priced in September and scarce and high-priced in the spring?

The reason is that the suppliers of coffee, in deciding how much to sell in September, are aware of the fact that there will be a demand for coffee next May. These suppliers probably know a lot more about our coffee-drinking habits than we do. Though we consumers may not even be aware of our drinking habits, the suppliers are balancing our demand for coffee in the future against our demand for coffee right now. The motivation for the producers is, of course, profit. Those suppliers who make good guesses about the demand for coffee in the future are rewarded with more profit. Those who make bad guesses are penalized with losses. The free market, then, furnishes suppliers with powerful incentives to give us consumers precisely what we want — the ability to buy as much coffee as we like for roughly the same price at any time of the year.

The decision on the part of business firms to make capital investments is very similar to the decision to hold back on coffee sales in the current period. Firms that make capital investments today are betting on a consumer demand for their products in the future. Such firms rarely *ask* consumers about their future demands. The reason is that, like the suppliers of coffee, the producers can often predict more accurately what consumers will want in the future than the consumers themselves.

Once private decision making is replaced by public decision making, however, things are very different. In a democracy, voters are forced to make decisions themselves on how much capital spending there should be. And precisely because voters are "rationally" ignorant about such matters, these are decisions that they are ill-prepared to make. Socialism in the coffee market, for example, might work something like this: candidates competing for office in September might woo the voters by promising lower and lower prices for coffee. Since the voters are uninformed about the future consequences of a low price of coffee today, they are naturally attracted to the candidate who promises the lowest price.

But if all the coffee is gobbled up in the fall at bargain basement prices, won't that mean that none will be left in the spring? And if that happens, won't the voters turn their wrath on the politician who created such a disaster? Perhaps. But in order for politicians to have good incentives here, they must anticipate that they will be around in the spring, and that voters will make the connection between the spring's disaster and the fall's political policy.

Herein lies the difference between the politician and the business firm. In a free market, with well-defined property rights, those who make decisions about capital spending are the very people who will reap the full benefits if the decisions turn out to be good ones, and bear the full costs if the decisions turn out to be bad ones. Business firms, therefore, have ideal incentives — even if they do not always guess correctly about what the future will bring.

The politician's position is very different. For one thing, since voters are usually ignorant about the connection between capital spending and specific benefits, the politician cannot look forward to realizing the full costs or the full benefits of his decisions. For another, the politician is not likely to be in office for very many years. This means that long-term penalties and rewards are largely irrelevant to him. Finally, the politician has no property right in his decisions. The worst that can happen is that he fails to be re-elected in the future. And this may be an acceptable price to pay for the opportunity to hold office today.

For all these reasons, then, democratic governments have a natural tendency to skimp on capital spending. It is probably no accident that Britain, one of the most socialistic of the major industrialized countries, has one of the lowest rates of capital formation in the world.

John and Sylvia Jewkes, two British economists who are long-time students of the N.H.S., have argued on numerous occasions that the lack of capital spending in the N.H.S. was solely the result of the political pressures just described. Successive Chancellors of the Exchequer, according to the Jewkes, skimped on "those items where the consequences in the short period would be least noticeable and least likely to arouse protest.[12] They go on to write that

> Governments followed the line of least resistance. They laid emphasis on those medical items which constituted pressing day-to-day demand, yielded their results quickly and with some certainty, made something of a public splash and conformed with the doctrine of equality. Conversely, they tended to neglect those items where spending would bring only slowly maturing results, where economy would not be quickly noticed and therefore would be less likely to arouse public opposition . . .

These were the conditions under which preventive medicine, new hospitals and medical schools, occupational health services and medical research were likely to give way to a free supply of drugs, of doctors' services and of hospital care. However anxious a government might be to take a longer view, its resolve was likely to be weakened by the pressure of immediate demands; and by the hope that easier times were coming; that perhaps next year defense expenditures would be smaller, or investment needed for other purposes would be less, or the national income would rise sharply.[13]

Administrative Controls

One of the most remarkable features of the N.H.S. is the enormous amount of decision-making power that has been left in the hands of doctors. By and large, Britain's medical community has escaped both the discipline of the free market and the discipline of government regulation. In the view of Michael Cooper[14], Anthony Culyer[15] and many others, the enormous discretion left in the hands of doctors is the principle reason for many of the gross inefficiencies found in the N.H.S.

In addition to the power of G.P.s and consultants, other producer interest groups also have obtained pockets of power and influence within the N.H.S. These include the hospital administrators, the junior doctors and the non-medical hospital staff. The complaint made again and again is that the N.H.S. is primarily organized and administered to benefit these special interest groups, rather than to benefit patients. As Dennis Lees puts it,

> The British health industry exists for its own sake, in the interest of the producer groups that make it up. The welfare of patients is a random by-product, depending on how conflicts between the groups and between them and government happen to shake down at any particular time.[16]

Government production of goods and services always tends to be less efficient than the private production of goods and services. Nonetheless, the N.H.S. could be run more efficiently than it actually is. Administrators could adopt well-defined goals for the N.H.S. They could assert more control over the various sectors of the N.H.S. to ensure that these goals are pursued. They could create greater incentives for N.H.S. employees to provide better and more efficient patient care. Yet these things are not done.

That they are not done is hardly surprising. Over 200 years ago,

Adam Smith observed that government regulation in the marketplace inevitably seemed to benefit producer interest groups at the expense of consumers. Things have changed very little with the passage of time. In the last ten to fifteen years, economic studies of virtually every major regulatory commission in the United States have come to the same conclusion: the welfare of producers is regularly favored over the welfare of consumers.[17] Why should we expect the N.H.S. to be an exception to the rule?

Are these phenomena consistent with public choice theory? At first glance it may seem that they are not. After all, consumers surely outnumber producers. So it might seem that, with democratic voting, consumers should always have the upper hand. If sheer voting power were all that were involved, this might be so. But two additional factors put consumers at a disadvantage: costs of information and costs of political organization.

In order to achieve any fundamental change of policy, voters must be informed about what kinds of changes they specifically seek. They must also be organized — at least to the extent that they can communicate to politicians their willingness to withhold electoral support unless their desires are satisfied. But as we have seen, information is costly. Organizing a political coalition is also costly. And the incentives for any single individual to bear these costs are extremely weak.

What can an individual voter expect to gain from a wholesale reorganization of the N.H.S.? His personal expected benefit from such a change might have a value of $50 or $100. If so, then $50 to $100 represents an important limit to his stake in the issue. In general, he will be willing to spend no more than $50 to $100 acquiring information and participating in a political movement to affect the change of policy.

But even this observation is a bit misleading. For the rational voter is sure to realize that a contribution of $50 to $100 of effort is such a small part of the total effort required that it is unlikely to make much difference anyway. In addition, if the political effort is successful, the voter will benefit whether or not he has contributed to it. So while the voter may hope that the overall effort is successful, he has an incentive to make no personal contribution to it. Since all consumers face essentially the same incentives, it is a small wonder that consumers have little political influence on government regulatory policies.

Producers are in a different position. Since they are working in the industry, they already possess a great deal of information about which policies are consistent with their self interest and which policies are not. The costs of organizing a successful political effort are also much lower for producers. This is so precisely because they are few in number (in comparison with consumers), and because their interests are far more similar. In addition, because the personal stake of each producer in regulatory issues is far greater than the personal stake of a representative consumer, each producer has a much greater *personal incentive* to contribute to political efforts that protect the interests of producers as a group.

Producer interest groups, then, ordinarily have enormous advantages over consumer groups in issues involving government regulation of their industry. These advantages appear to be more than sufficient to overcome their relative vulnerability in terms of sheer voting power. This insight was provided by Professor Milton Friedman almost twenty years ago:

> Each of us is a producer and also a consumer. However, we are much more specialized and devote a much larger fraction of our attention to our activity as a producer than as a consumer. We consume literally thousands if not millions of items. The result is that people in the same trade, like barbers or physicians, all have an intense interest in the specific problems of this trade and are willing to devote considerable energy to doing something about them. On the other hand, those of us who use barbers at all get barbered infrequently and spend only a minor fraction of our income in barber shops. Our interest is casual. Hardly any of us are willing to devote much time going to the legislature in order to testify against the inequity of restricting the practice of barbering. The same point holds for tariffs. The groups that think they have a special interest in particular tariffs are concentrated groups to whom the issue makes a great deal of difference. The public interest is widely dispersed. In consequence, in the absence of any general arrangements to offset the pressure of special interests, producer groups will invariably have a much stronger influence on legislative action and the powers that be than will the diverse, widely spread consumer interest.[18]

Public choice theory, then, predicts that administrative inefficiencies caused by producer interest groups within the N.H.S. will continue to be a permanent feature of socialized medicine in

Britain. There is no reason to believe, as many British critics apparently do, that this defect can be "reformed" away.

Why the N.H.S. Continues to Exist

Not long ago, an article appeared in *Medical Economics* with the heading, "If Britain's Health Care is so Bad, Why Do Patients Like it?"[19] That British patients *do* like the N.H.S. had been confirmed repeatedly by public opinion polls. The most recent of these showed that 84 percent of the British public was either satisfied or very satisfied with the N.H.S.[20] Almost all of the major complaints about the N.H.S. come from those who work within it and from outside investigators.

Why are British patients so satisfied with the N.H.S.? There appear to be two major reasons: (1) the typical British patient has far lower expectations and much less knowledge about medicine than the typical American patient; and (2) most British patients apparently believe that they are "getting something for nothing."

Comparing the difference between British and American patients, one doctor wrote that British patients "have fewer expectations" and are "more ready to cooperate unhesitatingly with the authoritarian figure of the doctor or nurse."[21] An American economist noted with surprise that British hospital patients, "far from complaining about specialists' inattention, a lack of laboratory tests, or the ineffectiveness of medical treatment, more often than not display an attitude of gratefulness for whatever is done."[22] Another doctor summarized the difference in British and American attitudes this way:

> The British people — whether as a result of different life philosophy or generally lower level of affluence — have a much lower level of expectation from medical intervention in general. In fact they verge on the stoical as compared with the American patient, and, of course, this fact makes them, purely from a physician's point of view, the most pleasant patients. The resulting service has evolved over the years into a service that would in my opinion be all but totally unacceptable to any American not depending on welfare for medical services.[23]

The expectations and the level of knowledge of British patients, however, is only part of the explanation for the popularity of the N.H.S. A more basic reason is probably the fact that most British patients grossly underestimate the amount of taxes they personally pay to finance the N.H.S. Public opinion polls have found that 60 percent of the British public believes that the entire cost of the N.H.S. is met, not from general taxes, but from the weekly payroll tax (called the "insurance stamp").[24] In fact, in 1972, when the opinion polls were taken, the payroll tax represented only 8.5 percent of the total cost of the N.H.S. Moreover, the worker's nominal share of the weekly payroll tax is only two-thirds — the remainder being nominally "paid" by employers. Although most economists believe that the employers' share of the payroll tax ultimately comes out of wages that would have been paid to workers, very few workers believe that.

A loose way of interpreting these results is as follows: most people in Britain believe that the total tax they pay to finance the N.H.S. is about 1/20th of what it actually is! Given this perception, no wonder the British public looks upon the N.H.S. as a good bargain.

Just how this perception of N.H.S. finances affects British attitudes toward what most Americans would regard as intolerable defects in the health service was vividly illustrated by the experience of Congressman Bob Bauman on a trip to England in 1975. Bauman had gone to England with a group of congressmen to examine the N.H.S. first hand. While there, he met a young woman with substantial facial scars received in an accident. Although the woman wanted plastic surgery for her face, she related, "I've been waiting eight years for treatment, but they tell me I'm going to be able to have surgery within a year." Yet when the Congressman asked her what she thought of the N.H.S., her reply was, "Oh, it's a wonderful system we have in Britain. You know our medical care is all free."[25]

It might seem that an enterprising politician or political party could win a British election by offering the British public a better deal. Why not tell the public what the N.H.S. really costs them, and then offer to return these tax dollars to the voters? Voters could then purchase private health insurance and other health services in the marketplace.

Would the average British voter be better off as a result of such a proposal? Undoubtedly, yes. But that doesn't mean that most voters would approve of the plan. For one thing, even if voters accurately perceived what the N.H.S. really cost them, they might not be convinced that the private marketplace could offer a better deal. For years, British politicians have told voters that the N.H.S. is the "envy of the world." And the public has been deluged with stories in socialist newspapers telling how only the very rich get good medical care in the United States.[26] In the light of so much negative propaganda about the American health care system, most British immigrants to the United States are usually amazed at how cheap health costs really are in this country.

For another thing, an enormous effort would be made to play on existing fears and suspicions by defenders of the N.H.S. These would include the highly ideological British trade unions, the thousands of N.H.S. employees, and a great many British doctors as well. Surprising as it may seem, the sagging morale and continual frustrations of N.H.S. doctors have not produced an enormous number of converts to free enterprise medicine. Perhaps a great many of them prefer the "protection" of a government bureaucracy to the rigors of competition in the free market. Whatever the reason, most of Britain's medical profession *supports* the idea of socialized medicine.[27]

The upshot, then, is that there is little hope for a successful political movement to radically alter Britain's health care system. Undoubtedly, the number of patients turning to private medical care and private medical insurance will continue to rise. But the N.H.S. itself will continue to be a permanent fixture of British society in the foreseeable future.

Footnotes

1. The two seminal works on public choice theory are Anthony Downs, *An Economic Theory of Democracy* (New York: Harper & Row, 1957); and James Buchanan and Gordon Tullock, *The Calculus of Consent* (Ann Arbor: University of Michigan Press, 1962). For more recent advances in the theory, especially as it applies to government regulation, see George Stigler, *The Citizen and the State: Essays on Regulation* (Chicago: University of Chicago Press, 1975).

2. Enoch Powell, *Medicine and Politics: 1975 and After* (New York: Pitman, 1976), p. 5

3. *Ibid*, p. 67.

4. Dennis Lees, "An Economist Considers Other Alternatives," in Helmut Schoeck, ed., *Financing Medical Care: An Appraisal of Foreign Programs* (Caldwell, Idaho: Caxton Printers, Ltd., 1963), p. 80.

5. Dennis Lees, "Economics and Non-economics of Health Services," *Three Banks Review*, No. 110, June, 1976, p. 9.

6. Joseph P. Newhouse, *The Economics of Medical Care* (Reading, Massachusetts: Addison-Wesley, 1978), pp. 85-7.

7. Joseph P. Newhouse and George A. Goldberg, *Allocation of Resources in Medical Care From An Economic Viewpoint: Remarks to the XXIX World Assembly of the World Medical Association and Commentary* (Santa Monica, California: The Rand Corporation, 1976), p. 9.

8. Mary-Ann Rozbicki, *Rationing British Health Care: The Cost/Benefit Approach*, Executive Seminar in National and International Affairs, U.S. Department of State, April, 1978, p. 17.

9. *Ibid*.

10. *Ibid*, p. 18. (Emphasis added.)

11. *Ibid*, p. 17.

12. John and Sylvia Jewkes, *Value for Money in Medicine* (Oxford: Basil Blackwell, 1963), p. 55.

13. *Ibid*., pp. 59-60.

14. Michael Cooper, *Rationing Health Care* (London: Croom Helm, Ltd., 1975), p. 73.

15. Anthony Culyer, "Health: the Social Cost of Doctors' Discretion," *New Society*, February 27, 1975.

16. Lees, "Economics and Non-economics of Health Services," p. 12.

17. A representative sample of such studies is contained in Paul W. MacAvoy, ed., *Crisis of the Regulatory Commissions* (New York: Norton, 1970).

18. Milton Friedman, *Capitalism and Freedom* (Chicago: University of Chicago Press, 1962), p. 143.

19. John J. Fisher, "If Britain's Health Care Is So Bad Why Do Patients Like it?" *Medical Economics*, August 21, 1978.

20. Annabel Ferriman, "Changing Role of the General Practitioner," *The* (London) *Times*, August 13, 1978.

21. Derek Robinson, "Primary Medical Practice in the United Kingdom and the United States," *The New England Journal of Medicine*, Vol. 297, No. 4, July 28, 1977, p. 189.

22. Rozbicki, *Rationing British Health Care*, p. 18.

23. Quoted in Harry Swartz, "The Infirmity of British Medicine," in R. Emmett Tyrrell, Jr., ed., *The Future that Doesn't Work: Social Democracy's Failures in Britain* (New York: Doubleday, 1977), p. 31.

24. Cooper, *Rationing Health Care*, p. 87.

25. Quoted by Lew Rockwell in *World Research INK*, March, 1979, p. 5.

26. *Ibid*, p. 6.

27. John Walsh, "Britain's National Health Service: the Doctors' Dilemmas," *Science*, Vol. 201, July 28, 1979, p. 329.

CHAPTER 11
Lessons for the U.S.A.

Drawing parallels between two different countries is always risky. Yet it is impossible not to be impressed by striking similarities between the politics of health in the United States today and the politics of health in Britain in 1948. One need only compare the public statements of many of our leading politicians with the public pronouncements of Churchill, Beveridge and Bevan over 30 years ago. Indeed, if speeches could be copyrighted, a good case for copyright infringement might be made.

Like the British in 1948, we now have a form of national health insurance — Medicaid and Medicare — which covers a large portion of low-income patients. And like middle-class Britons in 1948, our middle-class is feeling the financial squeeze. Not only are taxpayers bearing the ever-increasing financial burden of these programs through the taxes they pay, they are also watching medical prices rise precisely because of the programs. Enacted in 1965, Medicaid and Medicare produced a surge in the demand for medical care with no corresponding increase in supply. The result has been a dramatic increase in market prices. An early University of Michigan study concluded that between 1967 and 1968, physicians fees increased by almost seven percent more than they would have without the two programs. The price of hospital care rose by more than 14 percent as a result of their impact.[1]

Unlike the British experience, however, it appears that if a full-blown system of socialized medicine is adopted here, it will be adopted in stages. Stage I involves government controls over hospital spending — a necessary precondition for any program which removes all restraints on demand. Right now, most hospitals cannot expand their bed capacity or buy certain pieces of equipment without prior government approval.[2] Proposals before Congress will expand the government's authority in this area.[3]

Stage II involves a limited program of national health insurance. There are numerous such proposals before Congress and we cannot examine all of their particulars here. Suffice it to say that these proposals are generally intended to be "way stations" along the path toward fully socialized medical care. Most have built-in defects which ensure that they will not be acceptable in the long run. One proposal, made by the Carter Administration for example, would provide unlimited hospital and physician services to existing Medicaid patients — plus an estimated 10.6 million additional low-income individuals.[4] This proposal would clearly place additional financial pressures on the middle class, and encourage the demand for a fully universal program covering the entire population.

Strong pressures, then, are building for socialized medicine in the United States. Socialized medicine in this country will not be identical to Britain's National Health Service, but certain fundamentals will be the same. What can Americans expect from such a program? We can expect a lower quantity and quality of health care. Some specifics:

1. If health care were provided free of charge to patients at the time of treatment, the demand for medical services would soar and would far exceed the quantity that could conceivably be supplied. If American patients responded as British patients have, they would attempt to see their general practitioners four times as often as they now do. America, with its larger population, could look forward to hospital waiting lists which would exceed 2,800,000 patients.

2. Rationing by waiting is an inevitable bureaucratic solution to the problem of shortages in the health care market. Many patients would be waiting for years for medical treatment. Many of those waiting would be suffering chronic pain, and others would be risking their lives by having medical treatment postponed. A repeat of the British experience would mean 160,000 "urgent" patients waiting to enter U.S. hospitals.

3. The quality of medical treatment rendered would inevitably deteriorate. Doctors would spend less time with patients. They would offer fewer services. They would be less careful in the course of medical treatment. There would be fewer tests and fewer precautions to ensure the health and safety of patients. The ability of patients to protect themselves would diminish as the government moved to insulate itself from costly malpractice suits.

Recall that in order for British G.P.s to meet their heavy caseloads, they have all but eliminated the general checkup (which American patients customarily expect), and vaccination rates against major childhood diseases are at alarmingly low levels. As for the quality of care delivered in British hospitals, one comparison summarizes the vast difference between British and American health care: in 1970, 27 percent of all food poisoning cases in Britain occurred in hospitals. The U.S. Center for Disease Control reported not a single case of hospital food poisoning that year in the United States.

4. Political pressures would inevitably dictate the allocation of health care spending. Potentially life-saving techniques of medical care would be sacrificed to the type of medical care that makes a large number of people more comfortable. Recall that British ambulances make approximately one trip for every two persons in the country. Yet those same ambulances lack the personnel and the equipment to handle genuine medical emergencies. The N.H.S. spends millions of dollars each year on G.P. housecalls, but refuses to provide those same G.P.s with the diagnostic equipment American G.P.s use to treat non-trivial illnesses. Home visits by British nurses and health visitors equal about one-half of all British households each year. Yet thousands of patients die because of the government's refusal to purchase CAT scanners, pacemakers and dialysis machines.

5. Political pressures would also induce government officials to skimp on capital expenditure for the sake of spending which produces more immediate results. It is no accident that over 50 percent of all British hospitals beds are in buildings built before the turn of the century.

6. Precisely because of the increased costs to patients of rationing by waiting, because of the reduction in the quality of medical care, and because of the changing priorities in health care spending, voters would place a lower value on dollars spent on health care than they would if they were spending their own money in a private health care market. Political pressure would lead politicians to allocate less resources to health care than would otherwise have occurred. If anything, the average citizen can expect to consume *less,* not more, medical care under socialized medicine.

7. Government ownership or tight regulation and control of hospitals would be inevitable. Costly bureaucratic inefficiencies would abound. Recent bumper stickers on American cars have captured the heart of the matter — "If you like the Postal Service, you'll love socialized medicine."

8. Despite the claims of politicians, and even the best intentions of the suppliers of medical care, health services would not be rationed on the basis of medical need. Those who actually receive medical care would be those who are most adept at circumventing the barriers of non-price rationing.

9. Inequalities in the provision of health services would probably increase. Despite the egalitarian goals of many proponents of socialized medicine, the greatest hardships would be felt by the very poor. Not only does the evidence from Britain point to greater inequality under socialized medicine, recent studies of Canadian national health insurance arrive at the same conclusion.[5]

10. Like the Postal Service and the public educational system, the health care industry would become increasingly oriented toward the interests of the providers of health care services. The industry would be organized, administered and controlled not to meet the needs of patients, but to resolve conflicts among producer interest groups.

But perhaps the most important thing that Americans can expect will occur not after the introduction of socialized medicine, but *before*. Most people in this country probably believe that the medical profession will go all out in opposition to any form of socialized medicine. Don't count on it. Recall that, in 1948, the majority of British doctors did not oppose the N.H.S. on principle. In fact, they *favored* the idea of comprehensive, universal medical care financed by the state. Their only objections were to the particulars of the scheme.

Even in this country the political position of the medical profession has been ambivalent. After World War I, it looked for a while as though compulsory national health insurance was going to become a reality in this country. High officials of the American Medical Association praised the idea. Editorialists for the Journal of the American Medical Association called it "pregnant with benefit to the public." Only after they took a closer look at the particulars of the scheme did A.M.A. officials reverse their position. Particularly persuasive was the expectation that doctor incomes might be lowered, not raised.[6]

True, many members of the medical profession today can be counted on to oppose socialized medicine — not just on the grounds of self-interest, but also for reasons of principle. Many others, however, are likely to adopt the attitudes taken by their British counterparts over three decades ago. As an example, consider the comments of Dr. John Fisher in a recent issue of *Medical Economics:*

some form of national health program is exactly what we're heading into. What can we, as physicians, do in the face of the inevitable? We'd best concentrate our efforts, I think, not in opposing the concept but in devising the kind of program we can live with comfortably. It would have to be one that's good for our patients, of course — but it's up to us to make sure it's reasonable and fair to us.[7]

If socialized medicine is ultimately defeated in this country, it will be patients, not doctors, who will be primarily responsible.

Footnotes

1. Michigan Department of Social Services, *Health Care and Income,* Research Paper No. 5 (Lansing, Michigan: DSS, 1971).
2. David S. Salkier and Thomas W. Bice, *Hospital Certificate of Need Controls: Impact on Investment, Cost and Use.* (Washington, D.C.: American Enterprise Institute, 1979).
3. For a survey of effects of existing and proposed regulations of hospital costs, see Jack A. Meyer, *Health Care Cost Increases* (Washington, D.C.: American Enterprise Institute, 1979).
4. *Ibid,* pp. 32-3.
5. Cotton Lindsay, *Canadian National Health Insurance: Lessons for the United States* (Roche Laboratories, Hoffman-LaRoche, Inc., 1978).
6. A highly informative history of this early struggle is contained in Ronald Numbers, *Almost Persuaded: American Physicians and Compulsory Health Insurance 1912-1920* (Baltimore: John Hopkins University Press, 1978).
7. John J. Fisher, "If Britain's Health Care is So Bad, Why Do Patients Like it?" *Medical Economics,* August 21, 1978, p. 83.

The following books are available from The Fisher Institute

QUANTITY   TOTAL PRICE

_____ copy of FUNDAMENTALS OF ECONOMICS: A
PROPERTY RIGHTS APPROACH by Dr. Svetozar
Pejovich. The inclusion of new property rights concepts
updates the field of economics in this basic textbook for
beginning business/economics students and educated lay-
men. 258 pages. 51 charts and tables.

$11.95 (cloth) _____

_____ copy of TAX LIMITATION, INFLATION & THE
ROLE OF GOVERNMENT by Milton Friedman. The
Nobel Laureate has been called the most influential economist of this era. This new book will give you a broad picture of economic research and a fascinating overview of free
market philosophy. It is sound public policy material. 110
pages, 15 graphs, 2 tables.

$5.95 (paper) _____

_____ copy of LIFE IN THE SOVIET UNION: A REPORT
CARD ON SOCIALISM by Dr. Svetozar Pejovich. A na-
tive of Yugoslavia, Dr. Pejovich uses new and revealing
economic facts about how Soviet citizens are *really* living
— a far cry from the Soviet government's propaganda. 101
pages, 11 charts & tables.

$4.95 (paper); $9.95 (cloth) _____

_____ copy of THOSE GASOLINE LINES AND HOW THEY
GOT THERE by Dr. Helmut Merklein & William P.
Murchison, Jr. An economist/petroleum engineer and a
journalist combine to provide an historical and current
economic perspective of America's energy shortages — including an examination of the new "windfall profits tax."
140 pages, 40 charts & graphs.

$5.95 (paper); $10.95 (cloth) _____

_____ copy of THE NEW PROTECTIONISM: THE WEL-
FARE STATE & INTERNATIONAL TRADE by
Melvyn B. Krauss. Professor Krauss presents a clear and
essentially non-technical discussion of trade theory and
policy in defense of free trade. 117 pages, 5 charts.

$4.95 (paper) _____

_____ copy of FISHER'S CONCISE HISTORY OF ECO-
NOMIC BUNGLING by Antony Fisher. Fisher uses 5,000
years of economic history, logic, wit, anecdote, and a keen
understanding to show how the free market system works
best to improve every citizen's economic well-being. 113
pages of fascinating reading.

$8.95 (cloth); $2.95 (paper) _____

Please add $1.00 **PER BOOK** for postage & handling* .... $_____
(Plus 50¢ per book state tax if buyer resides in Texas)
Enclosed is my payment in full of .... $_____
Name_____

Title_____Company_____

Address_____

City_____State_____Zip_____

Please send information about the Fisher Institute ☐
*Prepaid orders shipped postage free